MY OWN DOUBLE HEART BYPASS OPERATION AUTOBIOGRAPHY

DOUGLAS COX

UPFRONT PUBLISHING
PETERBOROUGH, ENGLAND

Douglas Cox

MY OWN DOUBLE HEART BYPASS OPERATION
AUTOBIOGRAPHY
Copyright © Douglas Cox 2008

ISBN 978-184426-501-5

First published 2008 by
UPFRONT PUBLISHING LTD
Peterborough, England.

Printed by Lightning Source

Douglas Cox

My Own
Double Heart Bypass Operation
Autobiography

By Douglas Cox

Douglas Cox

Introduction

After my heart bypass operation, I continued on writing my other three books. It was late 2006 when thoughts began drifting through my mind about my operation. I had just recently had one memory thought drifted onto another memory thought, and on and on my memory thoughts went. I now scratch my head, I think to myself, I have a good true to the fact story to write here and that's how this story that you are about to read now was borne. Everything I have written is purely from memory. I never wrote anything down at the time of it all happening. I didn't know I was going to write a story about it. I recalled all what the hospital staff had told me at the time of it all happening; such people as the nurses, doctors, anaesthetist, cardiologist, heart surgeon etc etc. I was always asking them questions about what they were doing and why they were doing it, always putting my nose in maybe when I should have kept my nose out, but it all paid off in the end and you can now read my actual story of how it all happened.

My natural way with people is always to bring out the best of humour in them; all the hilarious activities I write of are all true. To the fact, stories of what happened at the time, all purely brought on by me for my devilment of bringing out the best of humour in people. I have written my story in layman's terms, just like the patient sees it.

Douglas Cox

My Double Heart Bypass

My name is Douglas Cox. I am the author of my own autobiography which is called, "The Life and Times of a Country Boy by Doug."

With me being a writer I thought it may be interesting and knowledgeable for any person who may have the misfortune to undergo such an operation. I hope you enjoy reading my true to the fact history of my double heart bypass.

The best place to begin is right at the beginning. I had my heart bypass when I was fifty-six years old, which was in the year of 2005. But my early symptoms that something was wrong began quite a time earlier than that. I always prided myself as being quite reasonably fit, even though I smoked 20 roll-ups a day and drank about 20 pots "pints" of ale a week. All my life I have been a lad of the fields and countryside, catching rabbits and shooting and walking my dog long distances across the fields for hours on end, which filled my lungs with the finest and purest of fresh countryside air. As my carefree life passed on by, I eventually became a full-time rabbit catcher which I did for more than 20 years in the Yorkshire Dales. This is what my book I wrote is all about.

I would catch myself walking $17^{1/2}$ hundred feet up into the hills without stopping and without hardly blowing when I got to the top, and that's with 30 rabbits strewn over my back. So now you readers know the keep-fit lifestyle which I led, except for my 20 roll-ups a day and my 20 pint pots of ale a week.

Approximately about two years before my heart bypass, which was in 2005, I began experiencing all was not well. I remember I was at home one evening watching television. My sister, Ann, who I live with, and me were sat on the sofa, my pup which is my rabbiting dog were sandwiched between us. I began feeling a little queer and a little unwell; it was as if my body was being starved of oxygen, but there appeared to be plenty of oxygen in the living room where we all sat. Ann said she felt okay and I could see pup was okay as she lay snoring her head off sandwiched between us. I had to get up and go and sit outside on the doorstep to get a breath of fresh air. As I sat there I began feeling very poorly; it was evening outside and was bitterly cold. I just sat there on the doorstep with just my thin cotton t-shirt on. I felt that poorly wild horses couldn't have pulled me up off that doorstep; sweat was pouring down my face and dripping off my chin, my t-shirt was wringing wet with sweat, my bowels inside of me liquefied, but I feared to get up and go to the toilet. I was feeling that unwell. After about five minutes had passed on by, I began feeling much better. I then had to go to the toilet; I had the "runs" terribly badly, and then after that I was champion again. My well being all came back again. I still kept on thinking it was lack of oxygen in the living room.

Over the following two years I had about six of these spells of being poorly and feeling unwell. I got that while I would go outside, usually in the dark, I would lay on my back and then on my side on the freezing cold grass lawn. I would lay there feeling very poorly and unwell. I would be looking at the stars up in the heavens. I am sure I could hear Gabriel blowing his horn for me to go to him up in heaven, but I knew I had a lot more rabbits to catch before Gabriel took me. As I lay there on the lawn, my t-shirt would be saturated in sweat. It would be so cold outside it felt as though the beads of sweat were freezing to my face, but I still kept on sweating profusely, and each time I got these spasms of feeling unwell, they all only lasted about a good five minutes. I just shrugged it off and classed it as nothing; I never even told my family doctor about it.

As time rolled by, it was about the month of March 2005, I began getting pulsations in my left arm and pins and needles in my left hand and fingers. This concerned me a little. I have heard people in the past say symptoms like that is a sign there's something wrong with the heart. Putting this throbbing pulsating and pins and needles altogether with my spasms of feeling unwell and hot sweats which I had outside on the doorstep and out on the lawn, I was beginning to grow anxious. So I went to see my family doctor who then had me checked out by the practitioner's nurse. My blood pressure was normal. The nurse checked me out on the ECG monitor. What's ECG stand for? Is it ELECTRONIC CARDIAC GRAPH? Anyway, whatever, it stands for, the ECG results showed everything with my heart was normal. It showed I had a good healthy heartbeat and the ECG showed I had suffered NO strokes or heart attacks. I was told that a pulsating throbbing arm and pins and needles in my left hand and fingers could be a trapped nerve or any number of other things.

So, I went away from the doctor's surgery bright eyed and bushy tailed. I have now been checked out and everything says I am okay.

As time rolled by (it was by now early August 2005), I began getting what I called a belly ache which appeared to be just below or just under my rib cage. I would get this belly ache three or four times a week; it would maybe last for 15 to 20 minutes and then go away. While I had this belly ache it would make me feeling unwell and poorly. If I got this belly ache while I was in bed, I would get up and sit on the side of the bed while my belly ache passed on by. I would then feel champion and all well again. I never took the belly ache serious and never told my family doctor.

As time rolled by, it was by now the 19th of September 2005. When I got up out of bed that morning, I awoke with the belly ache. This time it did not go away after the usual 20 minutes or so; I had belly ache all day. By the time it got to four o'clock in the afternoon I was seriously worried. So I rang my family doctor's surgery to get an appointment to see the doctor. The receptionist says the nearest appointment I can have will be in two days' time. I say to her, "But I am poorly now."

She asks what my symptoms are. I tell her, "My left arm is pulsating and throbbing, I have pins and needles in my left hand and fingers, and I have a belly ache underneath my ribcage."

She says, "Doug, dial 999 and call an ambulance."

I say, "I'm not calling an ambulance; it's only a bit of a belly ache I've got."

She says anxiously, "Stay on the 'phone Doug, I will just go and have a word with the doctor."

After only a few seconds she got back on the 'phone. She says in a real worried anxious voice, "Doug, the doctor says you have to dial 999 for an ambulance straight away."

I say, "I'm not calling an ambulance, it's only belly ache I have."

She says in a worried shaking voice, "Hang on there Doug, don't go away, stay on the 'phone, I will go and see the doctor again."

She was back on the 'phone in seconds, she says, "Doug, can you make your way down to the surgery straight away, the doctor says he will see you straight away," in an anxious dithering voice. She says, "Make your way down slowly Doug, don't hurry or get excited."

So, on that, I set off down to the surgery. It was only a quarter of a mile down the road. As I am making my way down I'm thinking to myself, I don't know what all the fuss is about, it's only a bit of a belly ache I've got. Her anxiousness had by now rubbed off on to me. I was by now feeling really poorly as I went along the road. There were beads of sweat coming onto my forehead, people I knew spoke to me as I passed them by. I didn't want to know, I was feeling really poorly and sorry for myself. At one point, I didn't think I was going to make it, but I did.

As I walk into the doctor's surgery the receptionist who I was speaking to on the 'phone sees me coming as she looks through the window. She comes out to meet me. She's a real fusspot over me, she's just like an old mother hen. She puts her arm through my arm, she walks me over to the waiting room, she sits me down comfortably. She says, "Now you sit there while I go and see the doctor for you," and off she goes down the corridor towards the doctor's room. She no sooner disappears when she reappears. She comes to me, she says, "Come on Doug, the doctor will see you straight away."

She takes me and leads me through the doctor's door and then leaves me in the privacy of the doctor. I don't know who was the most anxious, me seeing the doctor or the doctor seeing me. He gets me sat down at the side of the desk, he takes my blood pressure, he says, "That's okay."

He undoes the front of my shirt, he then puts his stethoscope onto my chest, I see him screw his face up. I think what he hears he doesn't like by the looks of him. He takes hold of my wrist. As I look down, I see his thumb on my pulse, he's talking to me and counting my pulse rate all at the same time. He says anxiously, "I don't think you have had a heart attack."

When I heard those words that's when the reality hit me. This was the first time my heart had come into doubt. I still wouldn't accept there was something wrong with my heart. I am as fit as a fiddle, I think the doctor will soon realise that I only have a belly ache. But he didn't, he says, "The ambulance is on its way, I want you to go and sit quiet in the waiting room, the ambulance will be here soon."

I no sooner sit down in the waiting room when I see an ambulance pull into the car park. I see its blue light flashing. I still think to myself, the doctor's got it all wrong. I am fit, there's nothing seriously wrong with me. I get up and stride out well to the ambulance outside. There's a woman paramedic coming towards me. She says to me, "Are You Doug?."

I say, "Yes that's me."

She has a wheelchair with her. Before she has time to tell me to get in the wheelchair, I go past her and jump in the back of the ambulance. She comes racing after me saying that I am going to injure myself.

She introduces herself as Sally. I smile to myself over the top of my belly ache. I say, "That's one of my favourite girl's first names. I once had a dog called Sally."

That brought a big smile onto Sally's face. Sally straight away gets me laid on the stretcher in the back of the ambulance. She shuts the back door and the ambulance races off with the blue light flashing. The ambulance passes our house. I see my sister, Ann; she's just coming in from taking the dog for a walk. She stops and watches the ambulance go past her with the blue light flashing. She hasn't a clue that I am inside it. I say to Sally, "Stop the ambulance, let me tell Ann what's happening."

By now Sally has me strapped down onto the stretcher. The ambulance carries on regardless. Sally gave me an aspirin to take while I was in the doctor's car park. Now she's got my shirt front open. She's wiring all my chest up and onto a monitor. She's now got my trouser legs rolled up. She's now wiring my legs up. She's now taking my blood pressure. I tell her, "Sally, Sally, I've only got a belly ache."

She says, "Oh no you haven't, you've had a heart attack."

I say, "I can't have, the doctor's just told me so."

She says, "You have, lay still."

Sally asks if I still have belly ache. With all the fuss that was going off I had forgotten about my belly ache, but yes I tell Sally my ache had gone away. Sally says it's the aspirin that has taken it off.

So I had a heart attack between leaving the doctor's surgery and getting into the ambulance. Incredible; I never had any chest pains. I never even knew I had had an heart attack.

By now the ambulance had arrived at Pinderfields Hospital, Wakefield. It backed into the Emergency Department. I am quickly whisked out of the ambulance and taken to where Sally explains all the situation to the waiting medicals. Sally pushes me into a cubicle, gets me up and laid on a bed. She then blesses me with all her luck, gives me a big smacking kiss and off she went, drawing the curtain shut behind her.

As Sally left a doctor entered. He wired me up again just in the same places where Sally had just unwired me in the ambulance. He did his tests on what he had to test, had a few words with me as he unwired me, then left me laid there and drew the curtains behind him. I laid there listening to all the activity going on at the other side of my drawn curtain. I hear doctors rushing around. I hear newly arrived patients moaning and groaning. I laid there and waited and waited. I think I must have been forgotten about. By now I am gagging for a smoke. I roll off my bed and pop on my shoes. A quick peep round the curtain, everyone seems to be busying themselves so I head off the way Sally brought me in. There's doctors and nurses dashing here, there and everywhere.

I go outside through the main entrance doors where Sally had brought me in. I quickly rolled up and lit up. I see a young woman stood there in her night robe. She is doing the same as me, she's having a quick fag. I get talking to her, she tells me what she's in for. It was quite a lengthy story that she had to tell, so we both lit up another fag. She then asks me what I am in for. I say I have just been rushed in with the emergency ambulance. She asks what for, I tell her I have just had a heart attack. She looks at me aghast. She says, "Good God, it's a wonder you have enough breath to draw on that cig," and off she goes back into the hospital dragging me by the arm with her. As we are both going back up the corridor (there's still doctors and nurses rushing about here, there and everywhere), I hear a doctor say to another doctor, "I am looking for a patient called Douglas Cox. He's gone missing out of the cubicle."

I put my hand up, I say, "I am Douglas Cox."

He comes over to me, he looks all in frustration. He says, "You should have stayed put in your cubicle, I was worried you might have had another heart attack and been rushed away."

I am now put in a wheelchair and a nurse whisks me away. She tells me I am going to the Emergency Heart Ward. She tells me I am being admitted into the hospital for a period. I tell her, "But I am going rabbit catching tomorrow."

She says, "In your dreams you are."

She gets me to the Emergency Heart Ward, she hands me over to a pretty blonde nurse. Jo, she says they call her; she's now in charge of me. By now it's turned midnight. Jo lays me on another bed and draws the curtains around us. It was as busy here as the last place I have just left. There were doctors and nurses bustling about here, there and everywhere. There were several people attended to me there as I laid on my bed, each doing their different jobs and asking me medical questions and such. I hear patients moaning and groaning at the other side of my drawn curtains as doctors and nurses are tending to them. I am then left be and quiet to lay on my bed. As time rolled by I couldn't get much rest with all the hustling and bustling going on at the other side of my curtain. By now I was gagging for another smoke. I rolled off my bed and slipped on my shoes, I peeped around my curtain; again everybody around was busying themselves. I set off looking for a place I could sneak a quick drag. I come to some toilets, I go in, I look up at the ceiling, I see a smoke alarm fitted to the ceiling. I go inside a toilet cubicle and lock the door behind me, I open and lean out of the toilet window and light up my cig. The smoke detector won't pick up my cig smoke now as I am leant there puffing away. I look to my side, I see nurses. They are in their rest room by the looks of it. One of the nurses looks out of the window. She sees me leaning out of the window having a quick drag. I see her race out of her rest room and disappear. She's no sooner disappeared when I hear banging on my locked toilet door. I could see it was no use claiming innocence; I opened the door looking guilty. She's ranting and raving at me, she's pointing up at the smoke alarm, she's saying if that goes off I will have to evacuate the whole of the ward. I set off back towards my bed. She shouts, "Stop."

She has a wheelchair and in a raised stern voice she says, "Sit."

I'm stuttering and stammering trying to make peace with her; she snarls back and says, "Silence."

As we get to the nurses desk there's Jo there waiting to meet me. Jo says, "I am ashamed of you Doug, I put all my trust in you and you've let me down. I quickly shrug off all their troubles. I say to Jo can I ring my sister and tell her I won't be coming home. Jo hands me her mobile 'phone.

I tell my sister, Ann, I've had a heart attack. She goes into hysterics. I tell her to calm down, I'm okay, but I have to stay in hospital. After all the palaver I caused among the nurses on that Emergency Heart Ward, they then moved me onto another ward. I didn't get much sleep either. I no sooner got to sleep when I was awoken back up again. The morning shift nurses had arrived for work. The tea lady arrives on the ward, then the breakfast ladies arrive on the ward, then in pops the newspaper man, then in pops a nurse; she comes to my bedside. She's wiring me all back up again and onto a heart monitor. She's not looking happy as she looks at me dead in the eye. She picks up my hand and clips on a crocodile clip to the end of my finger. She says to me, "There, you're all connected to the heart machine monitor now. Now you can't sneak off for a smoke now, can you?," and off the nurse went leaving me stuck there on my bed. As I lie there feeling all sorry for myself I could see out of the window from where I lay. There was a pedestrians footpath which I could see. I could see the odd people walking past which are smoking as they pass by. The heart monitor was bleeping away at the side of my earlobe. I was feeling really down and sad and all sorry for myself.

Thank God I wasn't on that ward very long. I got moved onto another small side ward. There were only three beds in it. The other two patients in that small ward I got to know them quite well. In one bed at one side of me was Mohammad and in the other bed at the other side of me was David. Our small ward led out onto a larger ward, and all the patients in these two wards were in because they had something wrong with their hearts; it was a heart ward. Most of us, including myself Thank "God," were walking about patients,, not bedridden. I could run off to the toilet whenever I wanted, but there were some patients who were very unfit, due to poorly hearts; some of them would shuffle along very slowly to get to the toilet and be very much out of breath when they got there, others would have to be taken by wheelchair, but there were many nurses about and they were always very helpful. On my very first day in that ward I got myself caught smoking. I was in a toilet cubicle with a broken lock on the door. As I leant out of the window by standing on the toilet pot; it was daytime and I see the light on, I thought I will save electricity and turn off the light, it will save on hospital funds I thought. There was a long length of cord hanging down from the ceiling which came right down to the side of the pot. It's what I call a "lazy switch," or so I thought. I pulled the cord but the light doesn't go off. I kept on pulling and pulling but the light doesn't go off. As I am stood there on top of the toilet pot with my cig in my mouth pondering and thinking the lazy switch must be broken, I keep on pulling and snatching at the cord when all at once a young nurse comes dashing into my unlocked toilet cubicle. I don't know who must have looked more surprised, me seeing the nurse come dashing in with a cig in my mouth or the nurse who saw what she saw.

The young nurse was very understandable and didn't report me for smoking and she told me what I thought was the lazy switch was in fact an "Alarm Bell."

It's there for if a patient gets into difficulty while on the toilet; he just pulls this cord to alert the nurses. So I got myself caught right good and proper that time. In the time I spent on this ward I was a persistent illegal rule breaking smoker. I had the nurses doing war dances on the warpath after the persistent offender. I remember I was laid on the top of my bed one day,

Mohammad in the next bed to me says, "I am going for a bath."

A few minutes later I decide to go for a quick smoke. I go stand in the bathroom and have a smoke and a chat while Mohammad is having his bath. My cig now smoked, I leave Mohammad in the bathroom getting himself dried down with the towel. I go and lay back down on the top of my bed. I hear someone on the big ward. He's getting such a rollicking and a good dressing down by one of the senior nurses. Who should walk in our small side ward but Mohammad, the nurse behind him chewing blood as she's at Mohammad for smoking in the bathroom. Mohammad spoke poor English; he's cowering and stammering trying to tell the livid out of control nurse that he doesn't smoke. The nurse doesn't believe him. She says, "You don't kid me, I could smell your smoke."

So that day Mohammad got a good rollicking when it should have been me getting the rollicking. After that Mohammad always locked the bathroom door behind him so that I couldn't get in.

I can recall another incident that happened on that ward but on another day which were different nurses. I had been down to that same bathroom for a quick roll-up. I had leant out of the bathroom window purposely to keep the cig smoke out of the bathroom. These nurses around here have good noses. They can smell smoke where there is no smoke. When I had had my smoke in the bathroom that day, I see woman's hair lacquer spray on the shelf. I get it and squirt it all around the bathroom; the scented spray should now conceal the smell of any cig smoke. I then went and laid back down on the top of my bed and began watching the television. I hadn't been laid there for very long before in marches a mad crazy senior nurse. She looks at me and Mohammad dead in the eyes. Mohammad cowers under his bed sheets, the nurse in a terrible angry mood says, "There's been someone smoking in the bathroom again."

She goes over to Mohammad's bed, she lifts up his bed sheets and says, "Whoever it was has been trying to cover up the smell of smoke with hairspray."

She has a smell of Mohammad's hair. Mohammad is speaking some sort of Punjabi language as he cowers low. The mad crazy out of control, blood spitting nurse looks at me dead in the eye. She says, "If I ever catch the culprit he will be in serious trouble."

She backed out of the ward leaving me and trembling Mohammad to it. I say to Mohammad, "Aren't you due for a bath Mohammad."

He stays underneath his bed blankets.

While I was having my stay in Pinderfields Hospital I was under the watchful eye of Sue. She wasn't a nurse, she never wore a nurse's uniform. Sue would always be dressed smart in casual clothes. I don't know what rank Sue held amongst the many different hospital staff. She was kind of monitoring my progress. Sue came to me one day and sat on the side of my bed to have chat. She tells me that my cholesterol is sky high and at a dangerous high level of 8.5. She tells me that I am on 40mg of Simvastatin and that this should bring my cholesterol down to a more safer level. I ask Sue what's caused my cholesterol to be so high. Sue says there are a number of things that can contribute to high cholesterol; having an unhealthy diet can contribute. I tell Sue I have been a big fatty eater all my life; I would often eat big lumps of pork crackling and as my mother, Edith, would take out the Sunday joint from the oven, I would grab big pieces of fat from it, and even when I made a sandwich I would lay on the best butter heavily using a quarter of a pound of butter just on one sandwich. Sue says, "There will be no more of that now, you must eat a more healthy diet."

I say to Sue on the build up to my heart attack and also when I had my heart attack I had no chest pains whatsoever. Sue says, "Some people suffer chest pains and some people suffer other discomforts like you did with your belly ache."

I say to Sue, "I was reading my confidential file at the end of my bed. It says 'NEEDS SEEING URGENTLY'. What was that for?" I ask. Sue says that's when you were first rushed in with your heart attack down in the Emergency Department. You were showing serious signs and had to be checked out promptly. I tell Sue I was curious about my heart attack I had just experienced. I say to her my friend had recently dropped 'stone dead' with a heart attack. I ask Sue why it struck him dead and I survived my heart attack.

Sue gets a piece of scrap paper. She sketches a heart. She tells me, "More than likely your friend's heart attack must have struck him in a vital part at the top of the heart. You Doug, were more lucky. Your heart attack has struck you in a less vital position; it has struck you on the side of your heart and has only left you with a small scar. Sue carries on her conversation as she is sat comfortably on my bedside. She tells me that I must remain in hospital until I have been screened and checked out on a heart machine called an Angiogram machine. Sue says all this will be done as soon as possible and then hopefully I will then be able to go home.

Sue then 'upped' herself from my bed and off she went. The day soon arrived when I was to go on the angiogram machine. Mohammad and David were also due on the angiogram machine the same day. That morning all three of us were prepared by a nurse to go on this machine. We had to have 'No' clothes on, only a gown that fastened at the back, and we all had a pair of paper underpants to wear, plus a paper hat on our heads. The nurse brought in a 'laptop' into our small ward and this laptop showed us everything we wanted to know about the tests and screening the angiogram machine does. So all three of us now were all ready and waiting to go down in our own turns onto this angiogram machine. The nurse comes into our small ward, she sees all three of us laid on our beds all waiting for action. She says, "You're the first down Doug this morning."

13

The nurse had no sooner said that when in walked a hospital porter, he was pushing a stretcher. The porter loads me onto his stretcher and away we go. We meandered along hospital corridor until eventually we came to stop. The porter went and spoke to a nurse and handed over some files. The porter then came back to me and pushed me into a room. A chap came over and shook my hand; it's Mr Phil Batin. I met Mr Batin earlier in the week when he was doing his rounds around the wards. He's the cardiologist, he's in charge of the angiogram machine.

I am taken from my stretcher and laid on another bed-like stretcher. I am now laid under a machine; there's big circular cameras overhead. I see also overhead a television screen. I think that's a television for me to watch while the angiogram machine does its work on me. Mr Batin tells me that he will talk his work to me as he is in the process of screening me. Mr Batin is stood on my right side and a nurse is stood on my left hand side. Mr Batin lifts my gown and puts his hands up the side of my scrotum pouch. He tells me that he is making an incision into my vein so that he can introduce a colouring dye into my bloodstream. I can feel him working away down there but I feel no pain as he makes his incision. He must have numbed that part of my body. Mr Batin says, "Right, we are ready for action."

I hear the machine come into action. He tells me these big circular cameras rotate around as it is screening my body. The television screen is now on. I am looking to see what channel it's on; one of my favourite films might be on. Mr Batin says, "As the coloured dye is circulating my body, I will be able to see what's happening on the television screen. I think to myself so the television is not for me to watch a film on. I see the circular cameras above me start rotating around. By now the nurse on my left is right up by my side. She cosseting me and reassuring me. Mr Batin is giving her instructions. She's carrying out the instruction as Mr Batin tells her. I begin to get the collywobbles. The nurse sees me getting the collywobbles.

She grabs hold of my hand and reassures me. Mr Batin says, "Right, I am now introducing the coloured dye into your bloodstream. Watch the television screen Doug.."

He gives more instructions to the nurse. She carries out the instructions using only one hand, her other hand is gripping hold of my hand. Mr Batin says you will feel a hot burning sensation on the top and around my thighs as the coloured dye is inserted into my bloodstream. I feel a warm surge as it enters my body. There's more instructions to the nurse. The cameras are rotating around above me.

"Watch the television screen Doug," says Mr Batin. I look at the television screen, I see the coloured dye in my blood circulating through my veins. I see it circulating through the arteries of my heart. This will be telling Mr Batin if my blood is circulating properly. I feel a hot burning sensation on the top of my thighs just as Mr Batin said it would, and then as quick as it all started it all ended. Mr Batin says, "That's it Doug, it's all over now."

The nurse releases her tension grip on my hand. And to think I was getting the collywobbles; there was nothing to the angiogram machine. Mr Batin is back up the side of my scrotum pouch. He must be taking out the connections that he has had in my vein. He is now applying thumb pressure on that vein; he must be stopping the bleeding. The nurse goes about her business to the other end of the room. Mr Batin says in a quiet reassuring voice, "YOU NEED A TRIPLE HEART BYPASS AS SOON AS POSSIBLE."

I lay there dumbstruck! I couldn't believe what I hear, and that was the end of my screening on the angiogram machine. What devastating news I had just received. My mind was in turmoil as I was being pushed back to my small ward on the stretcher. As we are going along the corridor of the hospital, I am thinking it's unbelievable news, and to think only a short while earlier, before I had had my heart attack, I thought I was "as fit as a butcher's dog, as fit as a fiddle, I felt as strong as a bull."

That just proves how "looks can deceive," and I arrived back on my small side ward. I cannot say, "None the worse for my troubles," can I? I see Mohammad and David, they are now both dressed back into their casual clothes. The porter lays me back onto my bed. He tells me to lay still for a while. Mohammad and David tell me their appointment on the angiogram machine has been cancelled until the following day.

After I have laid on the bed for a while in comes the nurse. She tells me I can now get up and walk around the ward again. She tells me to try not to exert myself. I ask why's that then? The nurse explains Mr Batin stitched up my surgical incision with internal dissolving stitches and that they will dissolve into my body within three months. The nurse says, "Let me have a look then."

She goes up the side of my scrotum pouch, she inspects the situation with a lot of close-up scrutiny. I think she sees something wrong down there, it's taking her a long time to scrutinise the situation. She gets back up from her kneeling position. She says, "That looks okay."

I look at her, she has a big broad smile on her face which must have stretched from ear to lug. As she walks away she says, "Right, you can pull your gown down now."

I look at her again. She's blushing. I think, what's she seen then? The nurse goes on to tell all three of us. Different surgeons use different techniques when closing up the incision. Doug has had internal stitches in, he can walk around nearly straight away, but other surgeons may use a different technique for healing up the incision. They usually have to lay down for quite a long while until the bleeding stops.

As I am walking slowly up and down our little side ward and trying not to exert myself, just like the blushing nurse told me, Mohammad and David say, "You're looking troubled Doug."

In a choked voice I say, "I have to have a triple heart bypass and it's got to be sooner rather than later."

Mohammad comes running over to me. He's saying in poor English with a bit of Punjabi mixed in it, "Mister Dougie, Mister Dougie."

He has his arm around me, I don't know whether he was trying to mother me or smother me. Anyway, I pull myself together and come to terms with the operation I have to have.

Later that day, Mister Batin comes to see me. There's quite a few people with him. They must be his secretary and maybe his registrar, and who do I see at the back, it's my guardian angel, Sue. She's still keeping her watchful eye over me. Sue comes to me. She's just like an old mother hen over me, but Sue wasn't old. She was a pretty golden haired fair maiden. She says to me "I am sorry about the bad news you have received."

Mohammad comes running over again, there's tears running down his face and dropping from his cheeks, "Mister Dougie, Mister Dougie."

Someone shuts the curtains around my bed shutting out Mohammad.

Mr Batin shakes my hand again, just like a true English gentleman. He asks if I have got over the shock of hearing the bad news. By now I have renewed vigour and full of new found strength as I release my long handshake. I say to Mr Batin, "I am strong enough to fight to the bitter end."

Mr Batin says, "That's the right spirit I like to hear."

A long mourning voice came from the other side of the curtain, "Oh, Mister Dougie. Oh, Mister Dougie."

Mr Batin says, "It's not really such bad news. By the time we have finished with you, you will have new pipes to your heart, and you have a strong heart I can tell you. By the time we have finished with you, you will be a new man with a full healthy life ahead of you, so keep up the old pecker."

Mohammad mourns out again, "Oh, Mister Dougie. Oh, Mister Dougie."

Mr Batin says my arteries are badly blocked up and that I have been put on the 'ACUTE WAITING LIST'. He tells me that I will have the surgery at Leeds General Infirmary; that's where they specialise in such operations and that it will not be very long before I will be in for the operation. Another long drawn out mourning came from beyond the curtain, "Oh, Mister Dougie. Oh, Mister Dougie."

Mr Batin says, "Who is that damned man?."

I say, "Speak lower, he can hear you say my symptoms. He's coming out in sympathy with me."

Mr Batin says, "We now have you stabilised on heart medication tablets and that I can go home the following day."

And on that, Mr Batin shakes my hand again and the curtain's are opened back up. As Mr Batin is leaving, Mohammad sees me again, "Oh, Mister Dougie. Oh, Mister Dougie."

Mr Batin and maybe his secretary and registrar then scurry off out of the ward, maybe to get away from mourning Mohammad.

The following day I had got my marching orders that I was going home, and was I glad of that. I don't like hospitals, but hospitals are a nice place to come when there's something wrong with you. Mohammad and David were being prepared again for their visit onto the angiogram machine. My angel Gabriel, Sue, was getting me all prepared for leaving hospital. She gives me many different sorts of heart medication tablets to take home with me, enough tablets to make me rattle inside.

Mohammad and David are now on their way down to the angiogram machine. They both leave together. As they go, I say, "I will see you both when you get back," and off they go. As I am waiting patiently on my small side ward waiting for someone to tell me to leave, who should pop her head into my ward but Sue. She's just like an old mother hen around me. She says I must empty my locker before I leave. I say, "I have done."

She asks where it all is, I say, "Here," as I hold up a half full carrier bag. Sue says, "You travel light don't you"; not that light once Sue had piled all my heart tablets into my half full carrier bag.

Sue has some pamphlets in her hand. She says, "These are to tell you how to eat more sensible. Please stick to a healthy diet," and on that she pops them all into my half full carrier bag; it's not that half full now, its brimming over the top with everything she has popped in. Sue tells me that once I am home, "it will not be long before you receive your appointment to be admitted into the Leeds General Infirmary for your heart bypass operation. You are, as you know, on the 'ACUTE' waiting list so you will not be long. Sue carries on to say, "Before that appointment comes you will receive another appointment. This will be for you to go to the same hospital, the LGI. It will only be for a day visit. There will be quite a few people there who, like yourself, will be waiting for a heart bypass. You will all be told what to expect once you have been admitted into hospital. You will be told everything there is to know about heart bypass operations and that if any of you have to ask any questions, all your questions will be answered, and once that is all over, everyone who is there for a heart bypass operation will be checked out. You will be monitored on an ECG heart machine. You will all have blood samples taken from you and then you will all go and have an x-ray taken. All this pre-assessment is to ensure you are fit enough and well enough to have your soon to come heart bypass operation. Once all this has been carried out, which takes only about four to five hours, you will all then be free to go home. As we sit in my small side ward and Sue is telling me all this information, Sue gives out a small ladylike cough with her hand over the mouth, she moves a little closer to me, she says in a quiet voice, "I have heard along the grapevine that you have been creating total havoc among the nurses for smoking. I have heard you have been caught and suspected of smoking here, there and everywhere around the hospital."

Sue moves in even closer to me. She says, "Take these wise words from me, if you do not stop smoking now there's a possibility you will not have your heart bypass operation, you may be rejected just because you are a smoker."

Sue carries on to say, "I want you to STOP smoking Now."

And on those wise words I heard from Sue that day I did as she bid.

My marching orders had now arrived and off I went, now discharged from hospital. Mohammad and David still hadn't arrived back from their visit to the angiogram machine. I bid everybody farewell and good luck to those patients on the big heart ward. I tell them to give my best regards to Mohammad and David and I have never seen Mohammad or David again to this day. I am sure they wouldn't have got the same news I got.

My niece, Eva Taylor, took me home that day in her car and from being rushed into Pinderfields Hospital at Wakefield by emergency ambulance, I spent one whole week in that hospital, and to think I thought I only had a bit of belly ache, "Symptoms can deceive."

As I look back over my life, I have spent my fair share of time in hospital.

I can clearly remember another time I spent in hospital. It was a terrible accident that happened to me. I have always been a lad for rabbit catching and rough shooting; that's a lot of what my book is about. I was so rabbit crazy in later life I ended up being a full time rabbit catcher doing it for a living. I have written many true life stories about that in my book.

This incident happened way back in 1964 when I was only a 15 year old lad. I decided to go to see if I could shoot a few rabbits with my 4.10 shotgun. I will just describe to you what my shotgun is like then you will know what I am talking about. My 4.10 shotgun was purposely designed to be a poacher's gun, and I have done plenty of rabbit poaching in my life, I can tell you. My 4.10 shotgun, if you press a button the gun folds up into two. I can then slide the gun barrel down the inside of my sleeve and the butt of the gun lays close to my body, so now when my coat is fastened you cannot even tell I have a gun on me at all. I have even walked passed gamekeeper's and they are none the wiser of the gun I carry. The butt of the gun is called a skeleton butt. This makes the gun very light to carry. The cartridges it shoots are two and a half inches long and a half inch round. It is full of small lead pellets and when fired out of the gun it has a range of about thirty yards. So now you are in the picture of what my gun is like which I am out shooting rabbits with. My faithful dog, Bess, always goes with me when I am rough shooting. In fact, me and that bitch, we were never apart. She was my best buddy.

We were going shooting rabbits that day on the fields that surrounded my home. As I walk along the sides of the hedgerows its Bess's job to hunt around in the undergrowth and flush out the rabbits to my waiting gun. A woodpigeon comes clattering out of the hedgerow. It's only about 20 yards away as it makes its escape at the far side of the bushes. I take a quick snapshot at it as it passes a gap in the hedgerow, the woodpigeon crumples up to the crack of my gun, and Bess is onto it as quick as a flash. She retrieves it back to my hand, I put it into my big poacher's pocket inside of my coat. I like to eat woodpigeon when I get home. I will skin off its breast and slice the meat from the bone. I don't wash off the blood; this helps it to taste even better. I will lightly fry it in the frying pan. It tastes like beefsteak to me, finger licking good. I will give Bess one half of the breast and I will have the other half. We always share and share alike does me and Bess. After all, it was Bess who flushed it out of the hedgerow in the first place. I pat Bess and make a fuss of her to let her know she has worked well. I send her back into the undergrowth again. I break my gun and slot another cartridge into the chamber. I see Bess, she's hunting like hell. She has her nose tight to the ground. I can tell by her body actions she's upon what she's hunting. A quick burst of wing beats strikes up in front of her, Bess leaps into the air after it. All she gets is a mouth full of feathers. It's a big cock pheasant as it passes in front of me. It's just about within range of me. I quickly pull the butt of my gun tight into my shoulder. I line up the sights just in front of the whirring pheasant, I pull the trigger and the big cock folds up to the bang of my gun. As the big cock bird hits the ground Bess is there to grab it. She retrieves it back to hand. What a big whopper it is. We will feed well tonight, will me and Bess. My ferrets back home will have a share of it also. I put the big cock pheasant on top of the woodpigeon in my poacher's pocket.

I slot another cartridge into the chamber of my gun. I wasn't to know it at the time but this cartridge had my name on it. We now head off and come to a railway embankment. I climb up the embankment and start walking along the top. Bess is below me hunting. I see her tail start wagging. She's onto the scent of something. She disappears under some blackberry bushes. I am sure she is going to bolt a rabbit out of the undergrowth so I pull back the hammer on the gun. I am now all prepared to shoot if the rabbit makes a run for it. Bess loses the scent and comes back to me. We now carry on along the top of the railway embankment, it brings us to the signal box. Brian is the signal box man. He is my friend. I usually stop and have a chat with Brian. As we are chatting away this particular day, Brian is up above me as he leans out of the signal box window. I am below stood looking up at him. I have the butt of my gun resting on the ground and I am holding the top of the gun barrel with my right hand. As we are chatting away together, I have an itch at the back of my neck so I reach over with my left hand and give it a scratch. As I bring my left hand back it passes over the top of the end of the gun barrel. There's such an almighty bang from my gun, my arm flies up into the air from the power of all the lead pellets hitting it. All this was done at point blank range. I bring my left arm back across to me. I don't believe what I see. There's blood spurting everywhere, all my veins in my wrist were just dangling out. I see blood pumping and squirting everywhere from my shot up veins. I look at Brian, there's shock horror on his face. Brian turns and runs to the first aid box. He shouts back to me, "What do you want, an elastoplast?."

I could see Brian was going to be no use to me. So I slung my gun to the ground and set off running. I ran down the hill that led to my home. As I am running I look behind me. I am leaving a trail of my blood on the road. I look at my wrist, I see blood pumping and squirting everywhere from my dangling wrist veins. I knew I had to hurry to get help otherwise I will have no blood left in my body. As I run into my house at the bottom of the hill there's Mr Tomlinson coming up the road. He's a first aid man, he sees what has happened to me. He rushes into the house after me. He quickly puts a tourniquet around my arm, the bleeding stops, my hand goes as black as coal.

My father, Ike, was out at the time. He was a pig dealer, doing it for a living, and having more than 200 pigs in a yard nearby. He always had the work for two cars so there was a spare car in the yard. Mr Tomlinson puts me into the spare car and rushes me to the nearest hospital. It was Hightown Hospital, Castleford, where they rushed me into the Emergency Department. The nurses quickly gave me emergency treatment and I was left laying on a stretcher waiting for the arrival of an emergency surgeon. As I lay there I heard the sister say to the nurse, "Keep a close eye on him, he will be coming into shock soon."

The sister was right. Not long after she had spoken those words I began shaking violently. The emergency surgeon was rushed in by helicopter and he operated on me straight away.

The next thing that I knew about it I awoke in a hospital bed the next day. The surgeon that had operated on me introduced himself to me as Bell-Tawse. He tells me that I was lucky. He says if the gun had have shot me two inches further up my arm he would have had to amputate the lower part of my arm. He also tells me that he has been operating on me for four hours, and that most of that was spent digging out lead pellets lodged in my wrist. He gave them to me to keep as a trophy. There were 60 of them altogether; Number 5 shot they were. Bell-Tawse carries on to tell me that he has had to sew all my veins back together. Also the guiders in my wrist had been blasted apart. He says, "with the guiders being elasticated, when they were severed apart one half of your guiders sprang back to your fingers and the other half of my guiders had sprang back up my arm. I have had to go searching for them inside your arm so that I could pull them all back together and tie them all back together."

I spent quite a time in that Hightown Hospital with my terrible shotgun accident.

In the time I spent in the hospital my father got to know Bell-Tawse well and my father found out that Bell-Tawse bred pigs for a hobby, so with my father being a pig dealer they both got on very well, and over the years after my accident my father bought many litters of pigs from Bell-Tawse. I didn't get rid of that hospital either; over the years that passed by I had to keep going back into hospital for a series of operations as my hand and wrist were rebuilt.

It was also found out the reason why the gun had gone off in the first place. When I was on top of the railway embankment I said Bess got the scent of a rabbit. I said that I pulled the hammer back on the gun making it ready for firing. That's where I made my mistake, I forgot to take the hammer off to make the gun safe. So when I was stood chatting at the signal box there was an old piece of wire on the ground where I stood, and this piece of wire somehow snagged onto the gun trigger and pulled it and "Bang," I got the full shot, so that was other long spells I spent in and out of hospital. But that's not the be-all-and-end-all."

I can recall yet another time I spent in hospitals and here is another true to the fact story that happened in my life. It all happened way back in 1981. My left eye swelled up for no apparent reason known to me at the time. I didn't think much of it, but as the days went by the swollen eye got worse. People who saw me said that I have a bit of cold in it, but the swelling got worse. Another chap I knew saw me one day. He tells me, "That's no cold in the eye Doug, take my advice and go see the doctor."

So I respected this chap's wise words and went to see my family doctor. He gives me some medication to put in my eye, but when all my medication had been used up my eye was more swollen than ever. I was also losing my vision in the eye so I go back and see the same doctor. When he sees my big swollen eye I don't think he liked what he saw. He sends me straight away to the Emergency Department to be seen by an eye specialist at Pontefract Infirmary. I sat there in the waiting room, I waited and waited. There were a lot of people there waiting. I noticed some of them were looking at my badly swollen eye. By now it felt full of pressure and now swollen more than ever. I was fast losing vision in my eye. I don't think the people in the waiting room liked what they saw. Eventually my name was called, I went into a small doctor's room; the eye specialist was there.

When he turned and saw my left eye he instantly looked concerned. I don't think he liked what he saw either. He had one of them special eye torch lights in his hand. He shines it into my eye. I hear him mutter, "Good God" to himself, he's now shining the light deep into my eye. He's so close to me we are both now eyeball to eyeball. He looks anxious to me. There's another eye specialist in the same room as us. He's on one of those big eye machines. The eye specialist is sat at one side of this eye machine and he has a woman patient sat at the other side of this eye machine; she is sat there with her chin on the chin rest. My specialist says to the other specialist, "I need to use that machine now."

He tells the woman patient to get up. The woman begins objecting saying, "I am before him."

This big eye machine now vacant, my eye specialist sits me down in front of the machine. I hear the woman behind me, she's still complaining to her eye specialist. She's still saying, "I am before him."

My eye specialist ignores her moans, he's more intent on getting me onto this big eye machine. I rest my chin on the chin rest. The machine has some kind of laser light on it. This light is shone deep into the back of my eye. My eye specialist appeared to be growing more and more concerned. The deeper he scanned into the back of my eye, the more concerned he appeared to be. He moves in even closer with the light. He's that close it keeps touching my eyeball. I keep blinking, he tells me to stop blinking, but every time he touches my eyeball I blink. He gets angry with me, he reaches over and he grabs hold of my top eyelid and doubles it back over itself. He says, "There, you can't blink now can you."

He's now so close with the machine it's touching my eyeball constantly, and he's right, I can't blink now. There's a nurse busying herself in the same room as us. My specialist says to her, "Nurse, book an emergency bed straight away at Pinderfields Hospital, Mr Cox is coming straight in."

I was gob smacked when I heard those words. The woman patient who had been moaning and complaining says to me, "I am sorry, I didn't know you were an emergency case."

I tell her, "Neither did I until just now."

I was rushed away to an ambulance car. I was put onto the back seat and off we go. The driver puts his foot down on the accelerator; it's about ten miles to Pinderfields Hospital. As I sit in the back of the ambulance car I think I haven't had a cig for ages so I decide to light up. I was always full of devilment for smoking where I shouldn't smoke. I remember we were racing across a place called Heath Common. I see the ambulance car driver, he's got his nose up smelling the air, he turns his head back towards me. He says' "Are you smoking?"

He didn't need my answer, he could see a cig in my hand, he snaps at me saying, "You can't smoke in this ambulance car, put it out now."

So I go to put it out in the ashtray, the driver snaps at me saying, "No, don't put it out in the ashtray. If the boss sees it he'll play holy hell with me."

He snaps at me saying, "Here, give me it here."

He snatches my cig off me, he lowers the side door window, he doesn't throw the cig away (maybe he was litter conscious), he puts his arm out of the window and nips off the red end of the cig. The back draft of the wind blows the red end back into the car, the driver starts doing some sort of dance as he sits wriggling about in the driver's seat.

"Ouch," he's saying, "Ouch."

The ambulance car screeches to a halt. We are now right on top of Heath Common, the driver quickly jumps out of the car, he's doing some sort of war dance outside by the looks of him. He's now pulling his shirt out of his trousers, off he goes again, he's now doing a belly dance. The people in the passing cars are slowing down as they pass us by. They are rubber necking, they must think my driver is some sort of entertainer. It looks as though the entertainment's over now. He's tucking his shirt back into his trousers, he's now storming back to the car. He leans over the back seat, he's glaring at me, he's blood red in the face. I tell him he has some sort of blood pressure, he's chewing and spitting blood as he's trying to tell me something. I tell him to "Drive on, I am going to be late for my appointment."

We reach Pinderfields Hospital all safe and sound. Well, the driver isn't maybe, he might have a few cig burns on his body. The irate angry ambulance car driver gets me to the Emergency Department which is right against the Eye Clinic Wards. As I go in the entrance who should be there to meet me but the same eye specialist which I saw at Pontefract Infirmary. I think to myself, how has he beat us to this hospital. It must be my ambulance car driver dawdling about on top of Heath Common. The concerned eye specialist ushers me into a small eye clinic room. He has his back turned to me while he's doing something. He tells me to sit down on the big back rest chair. The eye specialist then turns towards me. I shake in my boots at what I see. He has in his hand the biggest needle I ever did see in my life. I say, "What you gonna do with that then?."

He says, "Don't worry, it won't hurt."

I don't believe him, but he does it anyway. He sticks the big pointed needle right into my eye, but he was right it didn't hurt. He tells me he numbed my eye at Pontefract Infirmary. As soon as the big pointed needle comes out of my eye, I instantly feel great pressure released. As the eye specialist is putting some drops into my eye he's telling me there's something mysterious at the back of my eye, and that I must remain in hospital until everything is sorted out and, on that, a nurse came and took me on to the eye ward and showed me to my bed.

There were two eye wards with quite a few patients in them. One ward was for the women and the other ward was for us men. As the days passed on by I found out there were quite a number of different eye specialists in charge of patients on these two wards. The eye specialists really put me through it, scrutinizing and checking my left eye. They say I have some sort of parasite at the back of my eye and whatever it is it's attacking the back of my eye. I ask how the parasite got itself in there in the first place. They say I must have got something onto my hands and I have put my fingers in my mouth or I may have picked my nose and the parasite has got into my bloodstream and gone to the back of my eye. The eye specialist put me on eye drops called Atropine. This is made from the plant Deadly Nightshade. I have to have these eye drops put into my left eye every four hours. The nurse would wake me up in the middle of the night to put in my Atropine eye drops. The eye specialist put me on many, many Steroid tablets. The nurse came to me one day as I lay on top of my bed, she had my steroids I had to take. The nurse says to me with a big broad smile on her face, "Are they building you up to a world champion or something."

I ask the nurse what all the steroids are for. She tells me they are to build up my strength so that my body can build up a resistance and fight against whatever it is that I have in my eye. While I was in Pinderfields Hospital I had the freedom to walk around the ward, but I also had to have plenty of bed rest. This was for my body to build up even more strength.

I was beginning to be known by the nurses to be a persistent smoker in bed. The nurses caught me smoking several times. One day I read my Confidential File at the end of my bed; it said several times caught smoking in bed. So I got myself one jump ahead of the nurses. What I would do, I would lay under the bed blankets, I would have my cig under the bed blankets to conceal the smoke. I would also have a glass of water under the blankets.

So now if a nurse unexpectedly came on to the ward, I would quickly nip my cig into the glass of water which would then instantly kill the smoke.

My friend Clive who was confined to his bed, which was next to my bed on the ward, was an alcoholic and while he was in hospital, the nurses were trying to "dry" him out, free him from alcohol sort of thing.

Clive became aware of the nurses' tactics, so got himself some vodka which had no smell of alcohol and was clear, so it looks just like water.

Clive knew he mustn't let the nurses see his bottle of vodka which he kept hidden underneath all of his clothes in his cabinet locker at the side of his bed.

One day Clive decided he was going to have a right go at his vodka, let himself go a bit, so instead of him having to rummage about getting his vodka out of his cabinet each time he wanted to top up his glass, Clive emptied all his water out of his water jug and poured it all into his urine bottle which he used to have a pee in while he was confined to bed.

Clive then poured his full bottle of vodka into his water jug. Now his jug full of water is, in fact, a jug full of vodka and all went fine. The nurses were none the wiser; all the nurses saw was that Clive was drinking plenty of water.

So on this day, Clive and I were both laying in our beds busily chatting away, me with my cig lit under the bed blankets with my glass of water there at the ready, and Clive laid there merrily drinking away at his vodka, when a nurse should walk into the ward. She had a wheelchair with her and told Clive the doctor wanted to see him, and off Clive went in the wheelchair and disappeared out of the ward with the nurse.

Clive had no sooner disappeared when in walked a cleaning lady, who started emptying all the water jugs. She got Clive's water jug which she thought was full of water and she poured it all into a slop bucket, along with his full glass of what she thought was also water.

I was laid there gobsmacked as I watched her, but there was nothing I could do about it.

The cleaning lady emptied all the water jugs on the ward and off she went out of the ward with all the slopped-out water and Clive's preciously secreted vodka.

Now that it was all quiet again on the ward, I lit up another cig and smoked it while I lay under my blankets.

As I lay there puffing away at my cig. I hear raised voices approaching the ward, so I quickly nipped my cig into my glass of water and I lay there looking all innocent. I heard a woman's voice saying loudly, "You are drunk Clive, I know you are, I can tell you are."

I hear Clive pleading to her saying, "I am not drunk, then have a smell at my breath if you don't believe me," and in came the nurse into the ward pushing Clive along in the wheelchair. The nurse is playing holy hell with Clive for being drunk as she is putting him back into his bed. The nurse is struggling to get Clive into bed. He's so drunk, he's wobbling about like a paper necked Donkey. Clive sees his water jug missing from the top of his cabinet. Clive shrieks out, "Oh, my water jugs gone, nurse, someone's taken all my water."

Clive turns sharply in his anxiousness, he knocks the nurse scuttling across the cabinet, the cabinet topples over and the door flies open and out rolls his empty bottle of Vodka. The nurse continues her tumbling fall and crashes bang on top of me with all her weight. All the cig smoke which was trapped under my bed blankets all puffed out as the nurse lays across me. I must have looked a picture of guilt. I was shrouded in a thick cloud of cig smoke. As I look over the top of the nurse who's sprawled across the top of me, who should I see but the sister of our ward. She has Clive's empty bottle of Vodka at her feet. She looks terribly angry, she looks to be fuming. There's blood and snot coming down from her nose. The sister can hardly see me and the nurse on my bed for cig smoke. Clive's whimpering away saying, "It's not my fault, it's Douglas's fault," and we both got the biggest rollockings of our lives that day from the sister. We were both caught fair and square and both together. The sister had me and Clive separated. I was put into another bed at the top of the ward, as far apart as possible. The fuming outraged Devil possessed sister deemed me and Clive of encouraging each other to break the hospital rules.

After about a week of staying in Pinderfields Hospital at Wakefield, I got my orders that I could go home. The eye specialist tells me that he now has my eye stabilised. He tells me I must keep on putting my eye drops into my eye four times a day. The Atropine, Deadly Nightshade, should in the near future take control and eradicate the parasite which was attacking the back of my eye. So when I would go to bed at home I would have to put the alarm clock on to get me up in the early hours of the morning to take my drops. The eye specialist kept me under very close observation. I would often go to the Outpatient Eye Clinic at Pontefract Hospital. After quite a while of keeping up to my clinic appointments and keeping up with my eye drops four times a day, the eye specialist has me on the deep eye scanning machine. He says, "Good, God, the Atropine has not even touched whatever it is that's at the back of your eye," continuing on to say, "The Atropine will eradicate almost anything after three months. You must keep on taking the Atropine eye drops four times a day."

Eventually, after taking the Atropine eye drops for a further six months, the drops gained an advantage and eradicated whatever it was at the back of my eye. By now my eyes, BOTH OF THEM NOW, were really causing me great distress. I now had great big black floaters flying around in my good eye. The

31

eye specialist tells me not to worry, these floaters were coming anyway, they have nothing to do with the problem you have in your other eye. He says, "The floaters will not hurt you, you must tolerate them and learn to live with them."

I thought it isn't him that has to live with them. I ask the eye specialist what's caused my big black floaters to come in the first place. He tells me they are dead cells that are floating about in the jelly inside my eyeball. I also now had many problems with my other eye. Whatever it was that caused my problem it has now caused it to turn; it's looking in a different position to my other eye, it's called a 'Squint, Double Vision, Diplopia'. The vision in my bad eye, left eye, was by now very poor, but it still gave me double vision. With both my eyes put together and the problems each of them had, they were driving me insane. I was at my wit's end. They were sending me through purgatory, mental torment, great distress. But I still would not be beaten by all the problems, I fought hard to be strong.

I knew I had many more rabbits to catch in my life yet I kept on going to all my appointments at the eye clinic. They were every week and then every two weeks and then every month. Then a problem would arise and my appointment would then be every week again. But I was resolute, I would not bow and give in. I will fight these eye problems I have to the bitter end if I have to. Besides seeing the eye specialist regularly, I now had to see the orthoptist regularly. I was now trying to get my double vision corrected. The orthoptist taught me how to train my eye to put it back in its proper position. I trained and trained my eye for months on end, but it was all to no avail. All this time that was passing on by, I still had to keep on putting my Atropine into my left eye four times a day. This was to ensure the parasite in my left eye did not reappear. The orthoptist fitted me with 'prism' spectacles to correct my double vision.

To help matters along I had to have another operation, yet another stay in Pinderfields Hospital. The nurses dreaded my reappearance. They had fire smoke detector alarms fitted around the wards. They had fire buckets and fire extinguishers around the wards. I think the nurses were just being prepared just in case. The nurses were lucky, my friend, Clive, had gone home. The operation I was having at Pinderfields Hospital was to cut and retie my eye muscles around my left eyeball inside of my eye socket. That was another week or so I spent in hospital. My appointments at Pontefract Infirmary continued on and on. My Atropine eye drops continued on and on. Now my tied-up eye muscle was holding my left eye in a reasonable position, but that just made my double vision more closer together.

As time drifted on by I had appointments on top of appointments at the eye clinic. The purgatory and great mental distress continued on and on which led me to great despair. But I would not bow and give in. I continued on bravely and regardless. I knew I had many many more rabbits to catch in my life. My vision in my left eye continued to deteriorate; I could now only make out light from dark. The eye specialist now tells me I have a cataract on my left eye. He tells me it has formed with all the Atropine eye drops I have been taking and that I have to go into hospital for an operation to remove the cataract. So that's yet another stay in Pinderfields Hospital. After the cataract was removed, my eyesight in my left eye was now much improved. I could now see brilliant daylight. It was so brilliant my double vision was nearly intolerable. It was disastrous to my mental state. Most of the time I was completely disorientated; this caused great stress on top of stress on to my good eye. If I would have had a weak mind, it would have driven me to manic mental depression. But, luckily, I have a strong mind, I will fight to the bitter end if I have to. When my cataract was removed my eye lens was removed also. So, now my left eye could not focus. The eye specialist tells me I am too young to have an 'implant'; that's a false lens that they fit into the eye, so I am given an ordinary eye lens which I can put in and out when I wanted. That lens did not last long I can tell you. It made my double vision even worse than ever; it drove me absolutely bonkers. So, now with the lens out of my eye, it was out more than it was in. The vision in my left eye began to deteriorate with lack of use, my double vision was by now not as bad. As time went on by both my eyes began to settle. Even nowadays, (it's by now 2006) as I write this story, I still have slight double vision with my left eye which is by now very dim, but my prism spectacles which I wear all the time keep my left eye in a reasonable position. My right eye which is my good eye, thank God, that's as clear as a diamond. All the severe pressure and stress and strain it has undergone with pressures from my other eye. I can still knock a rabbit's head off with the .22 Rifle at 70 yards. It's a good job it wasn't this eye that suffered all the problems, otherwise my shooting days would have been over. The big black floaters which I had in this eye, they are much diminished by now, not a patch of what they were. The eye specialist did say I would grow accustomed to the floaters and he was, oh, so right. And now to the eye specialist's diagnosis. The eye specialist asks, "Do I keep horses."

I say, "Yes I do."

He says, "You must never touch a horse ever again in your life."

He continues to say I had got something off the horses onto my hands and whatever it was entered my bloodstream via my mouth or nose and went to the back of my eye and has caused a lot of damage. I tell the eye specialist of my life with horses. All of which I speak of here is all in my book which I wrote. My father Ike had two horse meat shops during World War II; he had one shop in Castleford and another shop in Leeds, and as well as him being a pig dealer he was also a horse dealer. A 'coper', that's the proper name for a horse dealer. My father bought many many horses to supply these two shops, but he also bought many many horses just for horse dealing. There wouldn't be a day go by without him buying or selling a horse, or buying and selling a horse-drawn flat cart or a four wheeled dray or a set of horse harnesses.

My father told me a story that happened before I was born. He was having a day off from his daily business of horse dealing, so for a bit of relaxation he went to Pontefract Horse Races. He tells me a big black stallion won the selling race; when the horse went under the auctioneer's hammer, the auctioneer knocked the black stallion down to my father, so even on his day off he was buying horses. When I came onto the scene in 1949, I grew up alongside of my father, always going with him buying and selling pigs and buying and selling horses. I remember him taking my mother, Edith, and me and three sisters to the seaside for a day out. It wasn't long before my father got talking to the man who owned the string of donkeys on the sands. My father ended up buying the full string of donkeys. My mother played holy hell with him that day. She tells him, "You're supposed to be taking me and the family out for the day, not buying the poor children's donkeys."

So, as I grew up alongside of my father, I grew up to be "Like father like son."

We would travel to all the gypsy horse fairs around the country buying and selling many many horses. We would travel up to Appleby Horse Fair in Westmoreland. We would travel by horse drawn 'Vardos' which are Romany Gypsy Caravans. We would take a whole string of horses up with us. On our travels up country we would meet up with other Romany Gypsies. We would set up camp with them for the night at the side of some lonely woodland. There would be many horses bought and sold around the campfire, horse dealing until well past midnight. Next morning the horses would be yoked up to the vardos.

"Vardi" is how they are pronounced in slang, once at Appleby. We would all get our positions and park up the vardis alongside the hedgerows as near to Appleby's Dealers Corner as we could.

There are hundreds of horses bought and sold at this annual event. There will be horses being trotted up and down the road on Dealers Corner. You will see the slapping of the hands as horses are being bought and sold. At the start of a day's horse dealing we will take a string of horses down into Appleby village and wash them in the River Eden. The horses will come out of the river looking as clean as a new pin. Then off they will go back up onto Appleby Hill and onto Dealers Corner. There will be big gatherings of people. We will have a string of horses there all tied up to the railings, all looking sparkling clean with them just coming out of the river. I will be on one of the horses riding it bareback just with a halter on its head to steer the horse with. The crowds of people will scatter as my horse goes trotting through them. The horses will be all geed up by some horse dealer cracking the whip behind the horse. My father will be somewhere in among the crowd of people. As my horse will be in a mad crazy trot, I will hear my father shout to me, "Bring that gallower in Doug."

Gallower is slang for horse. My gallower will be dancing on its toes as I take it alongside my father in the crowd. He will be in a mad crazy of slapping hands with some Romany Gypsy or traveller. The gallower will be sold. My father will shout to me as I am getting off the gallower he's just sold. I will hear him say, "Go pull that coloured tit out and trot that up and down the road."

Tit means mare. I will be on and off different gallowers all day long. By the end of the day my backside will be rubbed sore. I will see gypsy Benny coming across Appleby Hill, he will have three or four lurchers with him. Lurchers are fast running dogs. Gypsy Benny will have eight or nine hares strung over his shoulders. He will show the hares to the crowds of people. He will tell them, "My dogs have caught them, they are all good hunting lurchers. ."

Gypsy Benny will sell all his lurchers by the end of the day. By nightfall everyone will be washed and changed and down into Appleby village having a well earned pot of ale, and still the horse dealing is going off into the pub. There will be a secret fighting contest going off outside. There will be lookouts watching for the coppers coming. It will maybe be Gypsy Benny bare knuckle fighting out there. He's a good bare knuckle fighter is gypsy Benny. I have seen him take on two, sometimes three, men all at once and lick them all.

Appleby Horse Fair now over for another year, me and my father will now have more gallowers than what we went up to Appleby with. They will be all different gallowers all tied up at the back of the vardis, flat carts and four wheeled drays. I look at my eye specialist. He's sat there listening as I am telling him these horse dealing stories. He's sat there content with a cup of Rosy Lee in his hands. Rosy Lee is tea. I now tell the eye specialist how I think I got this parasite into my eye in the first place. I bought a gallower; it was very poor, no weight about it, so I gave it some worming powder. For days after that I would go through the gallowers droppings, 'shit'. I would be looking for dead tapeworms and dead ringworms that may have passed through the horse's system. I would go through the horse's droppings with my bare hands. I would never wash my hands afterwards. I could have put my fingers into my mouth or up my nose as I was picking it. That's more than likely how the parasite got into my bloodstream in the first place. The eye specialist nods in agreement. So that was the decisive decision of how my eye problem came to be in the first place. The eye specialist says, "I will have one of your books Doug."

He no sooner asks then he gets. A nurse has also been listening to my story. She says, "Can I have a book Doug?"

I nod. She says, "Can you sign it to my son?"

I nod. News soon spreads around the eye clinic, now there's more wanting my book. So, the eye specialist says, "I don't want to see you no more."

I say, "No more? Why, have you fallen out with me?"

The eye specialist smiles and says, "I mean I am discharging you from further treatment. There's nothing more that can be done for you."

I couldn't believe my own ears. It's become a way of life coming here and seeing all the doctors and nurses and the eye specialist had become a good friend.

All my problems had gone on for an unbelievable twelve long years. I kept all my appointment cards for some unknown reason. I counted up all the dates which I resolutely kept to, and from 1981 to 1993 I went to 86 appointments. Not a bad record I don't think, and to think right back to when my eye first swelled up. I was told that I only had a bit of a cold in my eye by my friends. But those shrewd wise words from another friend who told me to go see my doctor. So now you readers know my history of the number of times I have spent going in and out of hospital in my life, and now, here I am again.

It's by now the year of 2005 and I am now about to go into hospital for an Acute Triple Heart Bypass Operation. And all just as my golden haired guardian angel Sue had said, an appointment dropped through my letterbox. It says, I have to go to Leeds General Infirmary (LGI). We will be expected stay for only half a day and could I bring with me a urine sample and a list of all the medication I am on. That's no problem. I have all my medication and the strength of all the tablets memorised in my head. I acquire a urine sample container from my family doctor's surgery. The appointment day soon arrives and off I set to meet my appointment. I set off to Leeds on the public service bus. I sit next to a young man on the bus. He asks if he can cadge a cig off me. I tell him, "Sorry, I don't smoke."

I get off the bus at Leeds Bus Station. I now have a half an hour's walk to get to the LGI. On my appointment card at the back is a map to where I should go. The Leeds General Infirmary is one hospital which I have never been to. So, off I set following my detailed map. I set off up Eastgate; I know this part of Leeds well. It's an uphill walk as I go. At the top of Eastgate there's the Café Bolero where I would often call to have a strong pot of Rosy Lee and a bacon sandwich. As I am passing the café, Janet who works there sees me passing by.

Pretty woman is Janet, she's that pretty she can fetch ducks off the water. That's an old saying for a pretty alluring woman. Janet shouts to me, "I haven't seen you for a while, aren't you coming in for a bit."

I say, "A bit of what?"

Janet gives me a big radiant smile just like a breath of fresh spring mountain air. Her smile must have stretched from ear to lug. I tell Janet that I have recently had a heart attack and have now been put on a healthy eating diet. Janet loses her smile and frowns. I leave her stood there in the café doorway and off I head up Eastgate. It then runs on to the headrow and onto the Town Hall. This is where I have to start following my map. I have to turn right up Calverley Street, just before the Four Lions which are in front of the Town Hall. As I follow my detailed map, I am now passing by the LGI which is on my left. I don't want to be in this part of the hospital so I carry on along Calverley Street. This takes me past Calverley Street entrance into the hospital; it's called the Brotherton Wing. My detailed map says not here carry on. So I head on further up Calverley Street until I come to the top of the street. I follow my map and turn to the left and then left again, and there it is, the Jubilee Wing of the hospital. This is where I want to be.

I go into the hospital and to the reception desk. I show the receptionist my appointment and ask where I want to be. He says I want the fifth floor which is 'F' Floor. The receptionist directs me to the lift. As I am waiting for the lift door to open a dear old granny comes and stands by my side. The lift door opens, we both jump in. I am not in a hurry so I stand back and let old granny press the button to where she wants to be. I will just stand back and enjoy the ride. The lift no sooner sets off when it stops again. When the lift door opens old granny steps out. There's a chap stood there with a bright red boiler suit on. He ushers dear old granny back onto the lift. He says, "This is the basement dear."

I stand back and say nothing. Dear old granny presses another button. There's a loud speaker voice telling you all the time where the lift is going. The lift sets off. We are now passing 'B' Floor says the loudspeaker. 'B' is the ground floor. The lift carries on past 'C,D,E,F,G', and the lift stops. The lift door opens. We are now on the 6th floor which is the top floor. While dear old granny is muttering away to herself, saying this is not the floor she wants, I couldn't believe it. Another dear old granny appears. She looks exactly the same as the other dear old granny, but dressed in different clothes. The second granny says to my dear old granny, "I know how to work the lift, where do you want to be dear."

She tells her, she presses the button and off the lift goes. The lift appears to be going a long way for my liking. The loudspeaker is reeling off all the floors as we are passing them all by. I shut my eyes and have a rest. The lift eventually stops and the doors open. I don't believe what I see. It's the chap with the red boiler suit on again. He comes into the lift and while he's telling the dear old grannies which button to press, I sneak past the back of them and off the lift. I thought I will leave them dear old grannies to it. For all I know, they could still be going up and down in the lift. I head off through the basement; it's a bit dim and poorly lit down there. I work my way through different rooms. I come to some steps going upwards. It looks like an exit to me, so I go up them and through a door at the top. It brings me out into the hospital. Everything looks familiar. I have come out up the side of the reception desk. The receptionist I saw earlier sees me. He takes his cap off and scratches his head. He says, "How you got there then?"

I say, "You must have given me bad directions."

Before he has time to think anymore, I head off and disappear down a corridor. I pass by the lift I left the dear old grannies in. I see the light lit up where the lift is, I see it's still in the basement. No way am I getting onto that lift. I head off and take the steps up to where I want to be, 5th floor, 'F' floor. I go up all the steps all without stopping right up to the 5th floor, 'F' floor, and not blowing when I got there either.

Unbelievable, to think I am soon coming to this hospital for a triple heart bypass operation. I think to myself, have the doctors got it all wrong and there's nothing wrong with me in the first place. I now head on along the corridor, I get to about the point where the receptionist says I want to be. I see someone who looks like hospital staff. I show her my appointment letter and ask her where I want to be. She says, "You're Douglas Cox. We have been waiting for you arriving. You're late, everyone else is here and waiting for you."

I tell her, "I have been held up in the lift."

She ushers me into a small doctor's room. She asks me for my urine sample. I fumble about in my pocket looking for it, but I can't find it. I know it's in there somewhere. I pull out everything in my pocket. I don't see it. I give my snotty old handkerchief a shake and my urine sample drops out. The nurse picks it up carefully with just the ends of two fingertips and takes it away. It must be the urine sample she doesn't like. The nurse tells me to sit down on a weighing machine and she weighs me. She then tells me to take off my shoes and stand on the measuring machine. She now has me measured. She looks on her computer record, she sees my cholesterol is 4.2 from 8.5. She says, "That is excellent, your cholesterol when it was 8.5 was at a dangerously high level."

The nurse asks me if I smoke. I tell her that I am now a confirmed non-smoker. She says, "Very good Douglas."

The nurse says, "You are now on the Acute Waiting List for a triple heart bypass, you will not be very long before you are admitted into this hospital for your operation."

The nurse says, "Right, that's it. You have now been checked out, come with me."

We go into a corridor, there's a whole host of people sat there waiting. Another person who is hospital staff comes along. She says to me and the whole host of people who were sat waiting, "Pay attention everyone. I am your teacher, will everyone follow me."

So off we go down a corridor all following teacher. Teacher takes us all into a big room. There's a table there. There's trays of biscuits and buns, I see a big self-serving tea machine in the corner of the room. There's people hustling and bustling and talking everywhere. Teacher rattles the top of her desk with her ruler. She says, "Can I have everyone's attention please."

The room falls silent. Teacher says, "Please feel free to help yourself to tea and biscuits, and then could you all find a seat and sit down. I got my cup of Rosy Lee and biscuits and went to sit down by the window. As we are now all sat down, everyone now with a cup of Rosy Lee in their hand, teacher rattles the table top again with her ruler, she says, "Attention everyone please."

Teacher continues on to say, "All of you that are here today, are all due to have a heart bypass surgery in the near future."

I look around the room, there are about 30 people sat there, most of them had their partners with them. So teacher didn't really mean everyone was here for a bypass operation, just about half of them. I had come alone as you readers know. Teacher rattles the table again. She says, "Attention please."

I am daydreaming and gazing out of the window. I hear a voice saying, "Douglas, Douglas."

I look around. It's teacher, "Please pay attention, Douglas."

Teacher says, "Today I am going to tell you everything there is to know about heart bypass surgery. As I am speaking if there are any questions you may want to ask me, please feel free to do so."

Teacher has a type of cine camera. She is shining the film onto a white blackboard. She is showing us different pictures of the heart and showing us how the bypass surgery is carried out. People are firing questions all the time at teacher. Everyone's questions are being answered fully by teacher. I can't think of any questions to ask. I am getting more interested to the activity going off outside as I look through the window. Teacher must have noticed this. I hear the ruler rattling on her tabletop, "Pay attention Douglas."

Teacher has not fully got my attention. I feel something tapping me on my back. It's teacher tapping me with her ruler. She says, "Douglas, will you please pay attention to me."

Teacher goes back over to her white blackboard. Now teacher is telling us where the blood vessels are taken from out of our own bodies and surgically grafted to the heart which now bypasses the old blocked up arteries or narrowed arteries.

A vein can be taken from the legs for the bypass graft. If so, after your operation your leg may feel uncomfortable. You may have numbness or pins and needles around the scar on the leg, but this is quite normal, says teacher. You may also have swelling in the leg. A surgical elastic support stocking should help in this case. Teacher carries on to say another blood vessel which can be used in bypass surgery which is from the inside of the chest. This blood vessel is called the internal mammary artery. This artery is less likely to narrow over time than a vein graft. Blood vessels can also be taken from the arms and used for grafts. Someone asks teacher about the heart-lung bypass machine. Teacher says, "This machine does the work of the heart and lungs while the surgeon is operating on the heart."

Someone asks teacher if the heart is "stopped."

Teacher replies, "The surgeon can temporarily stop the heart."

Another asks, "How is the heart restarted again?"

Teacher says, "The heart starts to beat again as soon as the blood supply is restored."

Another asks, "What sort of anaesthetic is used for the coronary bypass surgery?"

Teacher replies, "General anaesthetic."

Another asks, "How long will I be in hospital after my operation. Teacher replies, "Anything between six to ten days. This depends on the person who's having the operation."

Another asks teacher, "Will I be able to go back to work shortly after my bypass operation?"

Teacher says, "It all depends on the person again, it's usually after about two to three months."

Another asks, "Will I be able to drive my car straight after my heart bypass operation?"

Teacher tells him, "You should not drive your car for at least four weeks after your operation, you do not need to contact DVLA after your heart bypass surgery."

The same person asks, "Will this affect my car insurance?"

Teacher answers, "When a car driver has had heart bypass surgery, they should inform their insurance company. If you have any problem with your car insurance policy, you can shop around other insurance companies, some of which are more sympathetic to heart patients."

A big fellow at the back says, "I am a heavy goods vehicle driver."

A woman at the front says, "I drive a public service bus."

Teacher replies to them both. She says, "Large vehicle drivers and passenger carrying vehicle drivers should not drive for at least six weeks after their heart bypass surgery. The drivers must let DVLA know about their heart operation. The drivers will have to have a satisfactory exercise test result before they can get their licence back."

Teacher asks, "Are there any smokers here?"

I decide I will have another cup of Rosy Lee while I'm there. I get myself some buns that are still on the trays. They're nice tasting buns these, they're homemade by the looks of them. As I am making my way back quietly with my Rosy Lee in one hand and my buns in the other hand, teacher is still speaking about smoking. She is saying, "If you have already had a heart attack, continuing to smoke doubles the risk of having another heart attack within one year. As I am passing teacher she says, "Douglas, are you a non-smoker?"

I tell teacher, "I am now a confirmed non-smoker."

Teacher replies, "Very good, Douglas. That's what I like to hear."

Teacher asks me, "Do you have any questions to ask Douglas?"

I say, "Yes, who's made the buns."

Teacher has a little titter to herself, all teachers' pupils give me a little clap. So, I now like asking teacher questions. I say to her, "I have another question teacher."

Teacher says, "Go on, fire away Douglas."

I say, "I am due to have a triple heart bypass in the very near future and I am told that it's Acute. What does Acute mean?"

"That's a very good question Douglas," says teacher. Teacher says, "When someone gets chest discomfort or chest pain it is sometimes difficult for the doctor to tell whether the person is suffering from unstable angina or having a heart attack, so if this happens to you your doctor may say that you have Acute Coronary Syndrome.

I now go back and sit by the window. I now have something else to say. I put my hand up into the air to get teacher's attention; teacher is busy answering other questions. I reach my hand high into the air, I am saying, "Miss, Miss, please Miss."

Teacher says, "What is it Douglas?"

I say, "Can I have your pupils' ears for a moment. Teacher allows me to take the chair and speak. I tell all the people sat there, I went to the dentist the other day and as I was laid on the dentist's couch the dentist was busy inspecting my teeth, he's always very pleasant is Mr Vincent. The dentist, he says, "And how are you Doug on this fine day?"

I tell him, "I have recently suffered a heart attack and that some time in the near future I will be going into hospital for a triple heart bypass operation. Mr Vincent is all ears to what I am telling him. He asks if I am on medication. I tell him, "Yes, I am."

Mr Vincent says that it is very important that he knows what medication I am taking. Mr Vincent goes over to his computer. I tell him all the tablets I am taking, he's putting them all down on the computer. He takes special notes that I am on 75mg Aspirin. Mr Vincent says that it is very important that I have informed him of all this. He says, "If ever I now have to pull one of your teeth out I must now take extra precautions against heavy bleeding from your gum."

He tells me the Aspirin thins the blood and bleeding occurs profusely. Mr Vincent says, "In the future if you are put on other medication, you must inform me so that I can update it on my computer."

Teacher says, "Thank you very much Douglas, that is very knowledgeable what you have just told us."

I again go and sit back down against the window. There's something going off out there that's causing me great curiosity. There's a couple sat against the window, it's David and Pauline. I have got to know them well while we have been here in teacher's classroom. David is a great big fellow in his mid-forties. He must stand well over six-foot tall. Pauline is very petite, much smaller than David and considerably younger than David by the looks of her. As we have been sat down together for a considerable time now listening to teacher. I have kept hearing Pauline whispering to David. She's been urging David to ask teacher a question, she keeps on saying, "Go on David, ask teacher now."

David eventually braves himself and puts his hand up. Teacher sees him, she says, "Yes, David. Have you a question for me?"

David starts stammering as he's trying to get his question out. Pauline's urging him on. She's digging him in the ribs with her elbow. She's saying, "Go on you big silly bugger, ask teacher now."

David blurts out, "Me and our lass here, we want to know if we can have leg over straight after my heart bypass operation."

Everybody starts jeering at David and Pauline for asking such an uncouth question to teacher. Teacher says, "Quiet please everybody. Please settle down. It's quite a sensible question what David asks."

Teacher goes on to say, "When you have intercourse it is important that you do not exert yourself David, you must let your partner do all the strenuous efforts. Pauline's ribbing David, she's trying to whisper but she's not doing very well. I hear Pauline saying, "What's teacher on about, what's intercourse, what's exert mean, go on you silly bugger, ask teacher what she means."

I intercept the situation. I tell teacher that her old fashioned language on sex isn't understood by David and Pauline. I tell teacher that in this day and age the word intercourse is now out of the window. It's not used no more, and what they call it now is bonking. There's tumult among the people. They are jeering and hand clapping. Teacher is shaking her head and blushing. David and Pauline are nodding their heads in agreement with me. They are saying, "That's what we want to know about, bonking not intercourse what teacher is on about."

So I say to David and Pauline, "When you're bonking on the carpet, you David must not do the hard work riding on the top. This will put pressure on your chest wounds and restrict your breathing. That's your job now Pauline, it's your job to do the riding on the top."

David and Pauline are now all smiles. Pauline says, "Now we understand."

Teacher interrupts, she says, "But you can't start bonking until four weeks after your heart bypass operation. Now the people are jeering at teacher for bonking about with the word bonking. I see Pauline, she is playing holy hell with David. She's saying, "I can't wait four weeks until after your operation. You haven't even had the bloody operation yet."

The activity going off outside gets the better of me.

I tell everyone to look out of the window, someone comes up at the back of me and leans on my shoulder. I look around, it's teacher leaning on me. As we are now all looking and

47

watching a party of 'Carrion Crows'. There's a sweet chestnut tree out on the lawn, there are many chestnuts on the lawn that have fallen from the tree. The carrion crows are gathering the sweet chestnuts and flying away with them. The crows are now on top of a set of traffic lights outside the hospital grounds on the main road. The carrion crows are now dropping the sweet chestnuts onto the road. Every time the traffic lights turn to green, all the cars are setting off and running over the sweet chestnuts. The carrion crows are sat up above on the traffic lights watching. As soon as the traffic lights turn to red, all the cars stop and all the carrion crows fly down onto the road and start eating all the smashed up chestnuts. When the lights turn back to green all the carrion crows fly back up again. All the carrion crows fly back towards us again as we are watching them from our windows. The crows are now gathering more sweet chestnuts from the lawn and off they all go again back onto the top of the traffic lights. Now that they have dropped all their chestnuts onto the road again, the crows are now leaning over and watching and waiting patiently for the lights to turn to red. They're all down onto that road again as fast as the cars stop. There's one of the Carrion Crows, he's dropped his chestnut and it's rolled safely to the side of the road. When all the cars stop he goes and retrieves his chestnut from the side of the road, he waddles back into the middle of the main road and places it exactly where the car tyres are running. All the time he is doing this he is half watching for the traffic lights to turn to green. He knows he's safe down there on the main road, while ever the lights are at red he's up before the cars set off when the lights turn to green. This time his chestnut gets squashed by the car tyres. Everyone is highly impressed at what they are watching. It feels to me that teacher's getting herself overexcited as she is standing very closely in at the back of me. I tell all the people and teacher, "The Carrion Crow is known to be one of the smartest, wisest, most intelligent birds of all birds."

Teacher says, "They are proving that to us now."

Teacher moves away, she says, "Right everyone, back to your seats, the show's over."

I tell the people who are still stood there amazed at what they are witnessing I tell them, "The Jackdaw is a member of the crow family and he's a wise old bird too. You can teach the Jackdaw to talk."

I hear teacher getting impatient, she's rattling the table top with her ruler. She's saying, "Will everyone please go back to their seats."

It looks as though no-one has heard teacher. So I carry on and say, "The Magpie that also is a bird of the crow family, he will gather anything that glitters The Magpie too can also be taught to talk."

There goes that ruler again rattling on the table top. It sounds as though teacher is becoming very angry with herself. She's now shouting across the room, she's saying, "Douglas, Douglas, pay attention Douglas. I am the teacher here. Come along everyone, please sit back down on your seats."

I let teacher take charge again and everyone goes back to their seats.

Now teacher has full control of her pupils again. It appears as though everyone has asked their questions. Teacher has told us all just about everything she knows about the workings of the human heart and heart bypass operations. Teacher now tells us all, "I now have a surprise for you all. For the next fortnight or two weeks, whichever way you want to look at it, you can now eat whatever takes your fancy. If you fancy fish and chips from the fish shop then do so. If you fancy a good old fashioned egg and bacon breakfast then do so. But do not please go over the top too much. Use a little common sense. This bit of what takes your fancy is to build up your body strength which will, in turn, help you through your soon to be heart bypass operation. Teacher carries on to say, "When your two weeks is up of eating what takes your fancy, you must all go back onto your healthy eating lifestyle and stick to your healthy eating diet for the rest of your life."

Teacher says, "Is all that understood loud and clear?"

We all acknowledge teacher's command. Teacher now tells us all, "Your lesson for the day is now over."

Teacher now carries on to say, "You now all have to go and be tested. You can have these tests in any order that they come. You will all have a blood test, you will all have an ECG, and you will all have an x-ray, and after all this we will then know if you are fit and well to undergo your heart bypass operation. After all this has been carried out you can then all go home."

Teacher carries on to tell us all, "You have an appointment card letter with you. Take your letters and report to the reception desk and you will then be directed from there," and on that, we all bid teacher good day and off we all go. Teacher gave us directions where the reception desk was. It was all on the floor below, 4th floor, E Floor. It's this floor we all have our ECG and our blood test.

I am at the back of the queue when we all reach the reception desk. I have been busying myself looking at the pictures on the walls in the corridor. There's one oil painting there of a village in the Yorkshire Dales. It really caught my eye; I have spent many years frequenting around this village and catching rabbits in the hills that surround this picturesque village. At the reception desk most of the people in the queue are being sent for an ECG first. I am sent for a blood test first. The 'blood sucker' (that's what I call the people who take the blood out of me), she gets me laid on her couch in her doctor's study room. I have my sleeve rolled up. She has a tourniquet around my arm. She tells me my vein is now stood up well. She turns to me. She has a big needle in her hand. I close my eyes, I tell her, "Don't let me see the blood she is taking out of me."

She says, "Come, come now, mummy won't hurt you."

She sees the sweat dripping off my finger ends in fear. I tell her, "I am squeamish and fear the sight of my own blood."

She carries on regardless anyway. I feel a slight prick in my arm and not much longer than a blink of an eye, she says,

"That's it, it's all over. You see, mummy didn't hurt you after all did she."

She puts thumb pressure on the point where she takes the needle out. She puts a bit of cotton wool over the puncture and tells me to hold it. She now holds the cotton wool there with an elastoplast and that's it, it's all over. There's nothing to a blood test after all, and to think I am squeamish. I am going to have my chest cut open soon. Not to worry I can brave it. The blood sucker now sends me off for an ECG, together with my appointment card letter in my hand. When I get there I see eight or nine people all sat there waiting for an ECG. I think to myself, I am in for a long wait here by the looks of it. I see a wooden holdall on the wall at the side of a door that goes into the nurses room where I presume the ECG is carried out. There's a notice at the side of the wooden holdall, it says, "Please put all appointment card letters in here."

There's quite a few appointment card letters in the wooden holdall already, so I pop mine in at the front of them all. Just as I am about to sit down to have a long wait, the nurse comes out of her room. She picks up all the appointment card letters out of the wooden holdall. I see her have a glance at them. She looks up and shouts out, "Douglas Cox, next please."

I think to myself, it's not such a long wait after all, and off I go into the nurses' room.

The nurse gets me laid down on her couch. I am now laid with just my jeans on. She begins wiring me all up. I have wires on my chest, wires on my arms, wires on my legs; I have wires on my body everywhere I look. I ask the nurse what the initials ECG stand for. She says, "Electrocardiogram."

It's a test to record the rhythm and electrical activity of the heart. The nurse started and finished the ECG all in a matter of a few minutes. She says, "I will just take all the wires off you and you can then get yourself dressed again."

The nurse hands me back my appointment card letter and off I head for my x-ray. As I leave the nurses room the nurse follows me out All the people that are sat there waiting for their ECG, when they see me they all start pointing. They are moaning and groaning and complaining about me. The nurse asks, "What is the matter with everyone?"

They all say, "It's him there, we have been waiting here for ages. We are all before him, he just comes along and walks straight in for his ECG. There's people right down the corridor booing at me. The nurse says to me, "You have put your appointment card letter at the front of the wooden holdall."

The nurse points to the notice board. It says, Please put all appointment card letters at the back of holdall. The nurse says, "When I picked up all the appointment card letters I saw your name first."

The nurse says, "You had better vamoose quickly before we have a riot on our hands."

So off I vamoose down the hospital corridor. I think to myself as I am vamoosing, them people back there are not very patient patients. They should be like me, a patient patient. The x-ray unit is on a lower floor, so off I head down there. There's hardly anyone waiting there when I arrive. So I sit down against the x-ray room door in the waiting room. I am now a patient patient all ready and waiting. The people who have just had their ECG done upstairs (the ones which I had just jumped the queue on), they keep arriving, sitting in the waiting room with me, and all in a few minutes they are called in and have their x-rays taken and then off they would go homeward bound. I am just left there in the waiting room patiently waiting. There's a chap, he keeps coming out of the x-ray room. He keeps on shouting more and more patients into the x-ray room. I am before all these people, but I am just left sitting there being a patient patient. My patient patience was beginning to wear a bit thin by now. So, the next time the chap came out of the x-ray room, I tell him I have been sat here waiting for ages. He says, "You must be going into the other x-ray unit which was next door to his x-ray unit. So, I remain sat sitting there patiently, patiently, patiently waiting.

There's more and more patients arriving, in and out of both x-ray rooms they would go. But, alas, I remain in the waiting room patiently waiting. After waiting ages and ages, the chap who I had asked earlier came out of his x-ray room. He says to me, "Are you still waiting?"

I don't have to answer him, I am sitting there as plain as day. He happens to notice my appointment card letter. It's half hidden underneath my coat. He says, "What's this then? You should have handed this in at the reception desk when you first arrived. So off the chap goes to the reception desk with my appointment card letter. He's back in "Two shakes of a lamb's tail."

The chap beckons me to go with him, and into the x-ray unit we both go.

The chap says, "Strip off to your jeans."

He's now pushing my bare chest on to the x-ray screen. He has now got me into the position how he wants me He says "Now hold still, don't move," and off he goes into his private little cubicle which is surrounded by glass panels. He says, "Now take a deep breath in and hold."

I hear and see a flash, the chap says, "That's it, all done. You can now get yourself dressed again and you can go off home."

My x-ray was all done and dusted all within a few minutes, and off I jolly well go homeward bound, which left me thinking to myself, I am not as patient a patient as I thought I was. Those other people certainly got their own back on me for jumping the queue earlier at the ECG unit. I now head off out of the hospital the way I came in. I sneak by the lift for fear of seeing them two dear old grannies. As I pass by the reception desk I bid the receptionist good day. He recognises me, he tipples his cap to me as I go. I am now outside the hospital again in the fresh air and off I go leaving Jubilee Wing behind. And that day out at the hospital wasn't a day at all; I had spent five hours there altogether. I get to thinking about what teacher had told us all earlier. What did she say? For the next two weeks we can eat whatever takes our fancy, but not to go over the top, use a bit of common sense. I remember I did go back to the Café Bolero on Eastgate that day. I did have one of my beloved specially made bacon sandwiches made by my special woman, Janet, and to top it all Janet threw in a large pot of strong Rosie Lee all buckshee and free. I did remember not to go over the top with what I eat just like teacher told us all. I knew in the back of my mind too much fatty material can build up within the walls of my arteries. There's enough fatty materials built up in my arteries already without me purposely adding to it. I did adhere to what teacher had told me, and two weeks' later I did go back onto my healthy eating diet.

After a short while of me being at home I did get a letter through my letterbox. It was my appointment to be admitted into Leeds General Infirmary for my triple heart bypass operation. The letter says my operation will be on the Monday, the 19th December 2005. The letter continues on to say that I will be admitted the day before Sunday, the 18th December 2005, so that I can be prepared for my operation.

The Sunday morning finally arrives. I have to be there for ten o'clock that morning. I catch the public service bus to Leeds City Bus Station; I travelled there alone. I didn't want to be molly coddled by a chaperone. I always travel light wherever I go, money in one pocket, toothbrush in my back pocket, that sort of thing anyway. All that I took with me that Sunday morning was a carrier bag that was only a quarter full.

I couldn't really come to terms with my heart problem. Here I was heading towards the hospital for an acute triple heart bypass. I couldn't really believe it. I felt as fit as a butcher's dog. I could have jumped over the moon I felt that fit, but at the end of the day the doctors are the experts. I made my way to the hospital on that Sunday morning going the same way as I did when I went to see teacher. I go in the same entrance to the LGI which is on Jubilee Wing. I am being admitted onto Ward 14, which is on the floor I know very well, Floor 5, Floor F. It was well signposted to Ward 14, so I had no reason to ask for directions. I walk along the hospital corridor and straight onto Ward 14. I go to the reception desk. I say to the nurse at the back of the counter, "Cox reporting."

The nurse looks at me, and then up at the big blackboard on the wall She says, "No, Mr Cox hasn't arrived yet."

I say, "No, I am Cox."

The nurse goes all into a fluster. She says, "We don't usually get patients coming in on their own, they usually have a big suitcase with them too."

She looks at my measly little carrier bag. She says, "Do you think you will be staying long?"

Another doctor arrives at the reception desk. He introduces himself as Jonathan. He says he will be in charge of me, and Jonathan leads me off down the corridor. He asks if I want a hand with all my luggage Jonathan takes me onto a small ward. There's only four beds on it. Jonathan shows me my bed. He looks at my measly quarter full carrier bag. He says, "You can put all your luggage in the bedside cabinet, if I can get it all in."

Jonathan introduces me to the other three patients on my ward and that was it. I was now admitted into Leeds General Infirmary for my acute triple heart bypass operation. Jonathan has something for me. He's now attaching an identification bangle onto my wrist. It says, Douglas Cox, 2-6-49, Leeds General Infirmary. I say to Jonathan, "What's this for then?"

Jonathan says, "That's for if you do a runner out of the hospital. The police will now know where to bring you back to."

Jonathan's now checking out all my details in my personal file that's hanging on the end of my bed. Jonathan is now giving me a thorough examination as I lay on my bed. He has a good listen to my heart. He says, "That sounds fine. We have all your other tests results from the 'Pre-Admission Clinic' you had recently."

I say to Jonathan, "What clinic's that then?" Jonathan explains, when I came onto this floor of the hospital recently, "You had an ECG, a blood test and an x-ray."

Then it dawned on me what Jonathan meant, it was that day we all came to see teacher. So that day was called a 'Pre-Admission Clinic'.

Jonathan now has his stethoscope on my back. He's telling me to take deep breaths in and out. Jonathan tells me he is checking my lungs. He says, "You have been a smoker up to recently, haven't you Doug?"

I think to myself, how does Jonathan know I used to smoke. News travels fast around the grapevine at this hospital by the sounds of it. I ask Jonathan about the operation I am about to have. Jonathan says, "Over 28,000 patients have coronary artery bypass surgery in the UK each year. Heart surgery has developed tremendously in recent years and, although a heart operation is Major surgery, techniques have advanced so much that it is now a routine operation. Jonathan has now checked me out and off he goes out of the ward. As Jonathan walks out in walks a nurse. I now have all my togs laid on my bed. I have my toothbrush and toothpaste, a towel, a clean t-shirt, a pair of socks and a clean pair of jeans. The nurse who has just come in is reading my personal files at the end of my bed. She is half watching what she is doing and half watching what I am doing. She says, "Where's all your other clothes?."

I say, "That's it, everything's here."

The nurse says, "Come, come now aren't you staying with us long?."

She asks me where my pyjamas are. I look vacant at her. She asks where my slippers are. As I shake my head the nurse leaves the ward Before I have time to put all my luggage into my bedside cabinet in walks the nurse again. She hands me a pair of pyjamas and a pair of slippers. She says, "You will want them for after your operation."

I could see by just looking at the pyjamas they were a mile too big for me, but I can't sleep in the 'noddy' like I do at home and, apart from a few more people coming to see me, that's about all I can remember of that Sunday when I was admitted into Leeds General Infirmary.

Monday finally arrived; the day of my operation. I was awoke early that morning. There were nurses here, there and everywhere. There were patients wanting bed pans and urine bottles. They were the patients that were bedridden and couldn't go to the toilet themselves. I was lucky. I was a walk around patient; I was for now anyway. In comes the breakfast ladies onto my ward. All three patients on my ward order their breakfasts and get their breakfasts and then the breakfast ladies set off to leave the ward. I beckon their attention. I say, "You've forgotten me."

The breakfast lady points out a notice on my bed. It says, "FASTING. NIL BY MOUTH."

A nurse comes onto the ward. She weighs up the situation. The nurse tells me I am second down to theatre that day, so it may be a few hours before my operation. She says to the breakfast lady, "Douglas can have a light breakfast, and then it's nil by mouth."

The nurse tells me, "After your breakfast Douglas, I want you to go and get a shower and get yourself prepared for your operation."

She shows me where all the showers, bathrooms and toilets were. There were many of them. There were many small wards just like mine and they all had toiletries to them. The nurse tells me to use any bathroom that is vacant. All the wards I now see are bustling with doctors and nurses, all busying themselves as they go about their duties. There were many different hospital uniforms they were wearing. I suppose that will be to put everyone into their own ranks. So, after I have had my light breakfast, which was just one slice of toast with "No" butter on (that's bad for the heart they tell me) it has to be a margarine sort of substitute that's "good" for the heart, I wash my toast down with a half glass of orange juice (they say the vitamins are good for my heart). I see that this place is a good healthy eating centre; nothing but the best to help keep a good healthy heart.

So, after I have had a good scrub in the shower I am now all spick and span and all clean and all that. Cleanliness is next to godliness or so they tell me. The nurse tells me this is how the surgeon wants me for my operation. A clean skin will help to keep out any germs or bacteria getting into my open wounds when he makes the cuts. I now go back and sit on my bed. I look at the notice over the top of my bed. It says, Mr Munsch, the heart surgeon. I think to myself, that's him that will be doing the cutting on me later today. I hope his knife is sharp enough. As I am sat there on the side of my bed pondering away to myself, in walks another nurse onto my ward. She says, "Would you be Douglas?"

She has to me what looked like a sharp razor in her hand. I think is she going to start cutting away at me now. I tell the nurse, "No, Douglas is not here. They have moved him onto another ward."

The nurse says, "Come come now, Douglas, don't be shy of nurse."

The razor was fair sparkling in her hand. She pulls of my t-shirt and my jeans. She gets her razor onto me and I sigh with relief. She wants to shave my hairs of my chest. I only have two hairs on my chest so it shouldn't take the nurse very long. But it did. She shaved me very thoroughly saying there must be no hairs there whatsoever. Mr Munsch will check the shaved area. He must not have any hairs in my wounds when he stitches me back up again. I tell the nurse, "Hirsute."

She says, "What' that mean?"

I tell her it means "Hairy."

The nurse, she's now shaving my legs.

"These are Hirsute" says the nurse. She's having to use two or three razors to shave that lot off. She says, "I have to make sure I shave off every hair right down to the skin I ask nurse, "Why are you shaving my legs?"

She says, "Mr Munsch, the heart surgeon, will be taking out one of your leg veins to do your heart bypass surgery."

I say, "But you are shaving both my legs."

The nurse says, "Mr Munsch will decide at the time of your operation which leg he will take the vein from."

I am now all shaved and ready for my operation, and off the nurse goes out of my ward, leaving me not as "hirsute" as when she came in. As I lay there on my bed inspecting where all my hirsute hairs had gone, I see three or four people come onto my ward. They have different hospital clothes onto the others I have seen. They look to me as though they have theatre clothes on. They are heading over to my bed. They are now introducing themselves to me. One of them shakes my hand and introduces himself as Mr Munsch, my heart surgeon. Now another is introducing himself; he says that he is the anaesthetist and says he will be looking after me throughout my operation. He asks me if I have ever had anaesthetics before. I tell the anaesthetist, "Yes, many many times before."

I tell him about all the operations which I have undergone, which you, the readers, already know about.

Mr Munsch notices I have been looking at my shaved legs. He says, "Let me have a look at them."

He is looking so closely I ask him if he wants to borrow my magnifying glass. Everyone around my bed gives a little chortle. The other people here must be members of the anaesthetist's and surgeon's team. As Mr Munsch is scrutinizing my shaved areas, he says, "The nurse has shaved you well."

I ask Mr Munsch, "Why it's just the inside of my legs that have been shaved?"

He points out my vein in my legs. He points to the bone that sticks out on my ankle. He runs his finger from there and up the inside of my leg. He goes up by the side of my calf muscle, up by the inside of my knee and up the inside of my thigh right up to my groin. He says, "That's the full length of the vein which runs up the inside of your leg."

He carries on to say, "I will have that out in a flash today and use it to bypass your blocked up arteries."

I say, "Well make sure your knife's sharp enough."

Everyone around my bed gives a small titter. By now the anaesthetist has his stethoscope on me. He says, "You used to be a smoker didn't you Doug?"

"That I did," I tell him.

"But not no more."

"That's what I like to hear," says the anaesthetist.

"Give me a little cough," he says, as he is listening with his stethoscope.

"Now breathe in and out nice and deeply for me."

"That sounds grand," he says.

"I have to check out your breathing before you have your operation."

The anaesthetist is now telling me the drugs he will be giving me in the anaesthetic room before my operation. He asks if I am allergic to any drugs. I say, "Not that I know of, only crack cocaine," I say in a little joke. Everyone around my bed gives a little titter to my joke. I tell him not to take me serious. I am not a junky.

Mr Munsch asks if I am feeling well. I tell him, "I have never felt better in my life. I feel on top of the world. I can still chase fair maidens around the bedroom and catch them."

Mr Munsch says, "We can make you feel better than that when you have had your operation."

Everyone gives a little chortle. Mr Munsch explains in great detail what he plans to do in my operation, telling me it's a triple heart bypass I am in for. I ask if it will give me much pain cutting me open and all that. The anaesthetist steps in and answers that question. He says, "He will make sure that my pain after the operation is kept under control. And that was it; the anaesthetist and surgeon say that I have checked out well for my operation. They say that it will be around midday when I am taken down to theatre, and, "We will see you down there

Doug, and on that they all left my bedside and disappeared out of my ward.."

I now lay back on top of my bed and drift off into a snooze. It was the sound of a squeaking wheel that woke me back up again. I look at the hospital clock up on the wall; it's by now ten o'clock in the morning. It's by now only two hours away from my operation time. What did the anaesthetist and surgeon say? I will be going down to theatre for my operation about midday. There's plenty of time yet so l lay back on my bed and rest. I am sure I can now hear two squeaking wheels or is it three squeaking wheels I can hear. The squeaking wheels get louder and louder as they come closer and closer. One of the squeaking wheels is that close now I open my eyes and look up. It's a nurse who has come onto the ward. She is pushing a drugs medicine trolley. She is now dealing medication to the patients in my ward. I now hear another squeaking wheel. It's coming onto my ward; it's the lady with a trolley full of fresh water jugs. This brought back old memories of my friend, Clive, at Pinderfields Hospital when he had a jug full of water or was that a jug full of Vodka. I hear yet another squeaking wheel coming. It's coming onto my ward; it's the newspaper lady with a trolley full of newspapers. She's a pretty woman is the newspaper lady. She asks me if I want a newspaper. I ask her if she has the Playboy magazine. She smiles at me and blushes. She says, "No, if you want that you will have to go to the newspaper shop yourself and get it off the top shelf."

It's getting rather hectic on my ward by now. There's squeaking wheel trolleys everywhere on my small ward. I think to myself, they must purposely have squeaking wheel trolleys to keep all the patients awake.

The nurse with the drugs medicine trolley comes over to my bed. She's putting a lot of medication tablets into a small plastic container. Yet another nurse comes onto my ward. She's coming over to my bed. She's handing me some clothes. She says, "Put them on and get ready for the theatre."

What a pretty nurse I think she is. She even wants to take me to see a show at the theatre. Yet another nurse comes onto my ward and to my bed. She hands me a tablet. She says, "Here, take that."

She tells me, "This is your Pre-Med tablet" and that it will help to relax me for theatre. I think to myself, I won't get much relaxation on this ward by the looks of it. The nurse with the squeaking wheel drugs trolley is now handing me a small plastic container. It has many tablets in it. She asks what other tablets have I been taking at home. I tell her quite a few different sorts. I tell her Aspirin to thin down my blood, Perindopril which I don't know what they are for. But the nurse tells me anyway. Simvastatin, which has crashed my cholesterol down from a dangerous level of 8.5 to 4.2. The nurse says, "Yes, that's right, I have it all written down here."

The nurse continues on to say, "We will prescribe your medication now while you are in hospital."

The nurse is now off out of the ward taking her squeaking wheel trolley with her. As that nurse walks out of the ward another two nurses walk into the ward. Wait a minute. There's someone else at the back of them. It's a cleaner lady. She has a big long brush with her. She's sweeping the floor as she comes onto my ward. The two nurses who have just come in, they are now making the beds. Here comes the lady with the water jugs to my bedside. I hear the trolley squeak squeaking along as it comes. She slops out my old water and replaces me a fresh jug full of water. As I thank her for the water she has to step aside; the cleaner lady is sweeping under my bed with her big long headed brush. She gives me a big smile that must have stretched from "ear to lug."

She bids me, "Good morning" as she sweeps past. As she is leaving I say to her, "Don't be wearing the brush out."

Her big smile is much broader now; it's stretching beyond from "ear to lug."

The two nurses are by now at my bedside. They tell me to get up while they make my bed so I get up and do as they bid.

They are putting fresh clean linen sheets on my bed. My theatre clothes are still there on my bed. The two nurses say, "You should have these theatre clothes on by now."

I wait while they finish making my bed. One nurse screeches out and pulls her hands back rather sharpish. The other nurse screeches out and does the same. I say, "Whatever is the matter with you two fair maidens."

They tell me, "It's the static electricity in the bed linen."

They tell me it's a regular occurrence getting an electric shock when they are making up the beds. As I turn and look to my side, there's another fair maiden nurse stood there. It's the same nurse that's going to take me to see the show at the theatre. She is looking at me with a determined look in her eyes. She says, "Haven't you got your theatre gown on yet?"

I ask her what time does the show start."

She says, "You will get bloody show, get yourself ready now."

I hear the two nurses making my bed. They are screeching out, "Ouch, ouch, ouch," but the two fair maiden nurses were determined and they did finish making my bed despite all the electric shocks they were getting. As they left my bed their work now completed, my other fair maiden nurse with the determined look in her eyes says, "Look at the time, it's midday, and you aren't even ready for theatre yet."

The nurse quickly draws the curtain around my bed. All the beds in the hospital have big curtains which can be drawn around the beds for privacy. My fair maiden nurse now has me right where she wants me, at the back of closed curtains. She whips my t-shirt off, she puts the theatre gown on me and ties it in a bow at the back. The nurse, she's now under my gown, she's whipping off my jeans, she throws my jeans onto my bed and grabs my paper underpants. She's now got her head up my theatre gown. She's trying to pull up my paper underpants. I hear another squeaking wheel coming. I hear it stop, a chap puts his head around my privacy curtain. He says, "Douglas Cox."

He then looks down and sees my fair maiden nurse up under my theatre gown The nurse has heard the chap speaking, she comes out from underneath my theatre gown. The chap is the porter who has come to take me down to theatre for my operation. He says, "I can come back if you're busy."

The fair maiden nurse gets herself up from her knees. She appears to be blushing to me. She pulls down and straightens my theatre gown. She says to the porter, "There, he's ready."

And on that the porter lays me on his trolley like stretcher. As I lay there, the fair maiden nurse says, "Just a minute."

She plonks my paper cap on top of my head. She says, "There, if cap fits wear it."

She says, "He's now ready porter. Take him away and drown him."

And off I go laid on the stretcher down and along the hospital corridors destined for the operating theatre. The squeak squeak of the porter's trolley was drifting me off into slumber, no doubt helped on by the pre-med tablet I had taken earlier.

We stop at some doors. Over the top of the doors it says, "THEATRE."

I think to myself, this is the theatre where that pretty nurse was going to take me to see that show. The doors open and I am pushed in by the porter. There's quite a few people in there waiting for me to arrive. I cast my eyes around, but I don't see that pretty nurse. She's stood me up by the looks of it. I am now pushed into another room. I now see my friend, the anaesthetist, the one who came to see me on my ward. He comes over to shake my hand. I ask him if he has sharpened his knife properly. I tell him that he can borrow my rabbit cutting knife, the one I paunch my rabbits with. I tell him it's razor sharp. My tongue is silenced; there's someone putting an oxygen breathing mask over my face. There's someone now telling me they are now giving me an anaesthetic drug injection and that I will only feel a slight prick. I no sooner feel a slight prick when I seem to drift off into wonderland. I am now aroused from my distant wonderland dreams by a distant voice saying, "Doug, Doug, wake up Doug."

I open the slits of my eyes, I see a golden-haired angel. She's looking at me straight in the eyes. I think to myself, I am having a deep romantic dream here. So I close my eyes. I hear the distant voice again. It's saying, "Doug, Doug, Doug, wake up darling, it's Michelle here, wake up."

I open my eyes wider this time. I see the golden-haired angel again. She's now that close she's touching the end of my nose with her nose. She's looking deep into my eyes. She's saying, "Doug, Doug, wake up darling, it's Michelle here."

I open my eyes wide now. The angel says, "Wake up Doug, don't go back to sleep on me."

I am now aware of activity going off around me. My mouth, it's wide open and it's all full of pipes. The golden-haired angel, she's stood there looking at me. By what a pretty angel she looks. She's smiling at me. It's just like a breath of spring mountain air. She's saying, "Are you alright darling, I am Michelle. I am looking after you through your operation."

By now I am fully awake.

Michelle isn't an angel after all. She's dressed in a nurse's uniform. She's now busying herself across the small room. I look around myself. I see more people; they are dressed in different hospital uniforms. They are busying themselves too. My mouth, what's all these pipes doing in my mouth I think. I see the golden-haired angel. She's coming back over to me as I am laid on some sort of a stretcher. She's saying, "Are you awake now darling" I can't answer that. My mouth is all spragged open with pipes. The golden-haired angel, she's now fondling my legs. I think to myself, I had better watch this angel. It looks to me as though she's coming heavy onto me. She's saying, "Doug, can you feel me touching your legs?"

I give her the nod the best way I could with all the pipes stuck in my mouth. The golden-haired angel, Michelle, she's now telling me to wiggle my toes. I do as she bids; anything to throw her off my scent. She's saying, "That's lovely darling," as she's watching my toes wiggle. The golden-haired angel, Michelle, she's now looking at me real close up, she's looking deep into my eyes. She says, "Doug, I am going to take some of these pipes out of your mouth."

She pulls one and then another. I feel them coming up my windpipe as she pulls. She's saying, "There darling, do you feel better now with all them pipes out?"

I can now speak to my relief. The golden-haired angel, Michelle, she's now trying to chat me up. She's now asking me what I do for a living. I tell her I am a rabbit poacher. She says, "Oh Douglas, poor little rabbits."

I say, "They are not poor, they are great big fat rabbits."

I tell Michelle that I have written a book about all my rabbiting days. Michelle says, "My son goes hunting. Could I have one of your books for him?"

I give Michelle the nod. She asks, "and could you sign it to him?"

I give Michelle the nod. Michelle says, "Right Doug, we are now going to move you on to the Intensive Care Ward," and off we go as I am being pushed along on some sort of stretcher. As we go along the hospital corridors I am still a little groggy from my operation, so I close my eyes while we travel along. I feel my trolley-com-stretcher stop.

I open my eyes. I am now in a small ward. I look around myself. I see no other patients in the ward. I am alone but I see nurses there all around. I see machinery around me. I have been that sleepy and groggy I now find myself laid in a bed. I never noticed anyone transfer me from the stretcher to this bed I now lay in. I now see tubes and equipment all around me. I see a nurse by my bedside as she is tending to me. She sees me looking at everything around me. The nurse tells me not to be frightened about all the machinery and tubes I see. She says, "This is all specialised equipment for the medical and nursing staff to use to record the action of your heart, lungs and other body systems. It helps them to monitor and keep a check on your condition very accurately."

The nurse looks at me and gives me a big smile and says, "All this monitoring we are doing plays an important part in the overall success of your heart operation."

I have some sort of mask over my mouth and nose, so I lift it up and thank the nurse for all that information. The nurse, she's trying to adjust the mask over my face. I lift it up again and ask her what it is. She says, "Don't be alarmed, it's only an oxygen mask. This is giving you a supply of oxygen and water vapour. It's a bit like steam for you to breathe."

I lift up my oxygen mask again. I say to the nurse, "Look at all these tubes I have stuck in me and all the wires that are connected to me. What are they all for?"

The nurse answers by saying, "The tube you have in the arm is connected to a drip which is dripping fluid into your blood. The other arm has a tube in your wrist. This is measuring your blood pressure. The pipes I took out of your chest earlier are called "CHEST DRAINS'. The surgeon has put these chest drains into your chest area around your heart. These tubes allow any blood which builds up in that area to be removed safely."

The nurse sees me feeling at the side of my neck. She says, "We have had a tube in your neck also. At that point, where you are feeling now, this tube was passing fluid into your blood circulation during your operation."

The nurse sees me feeling between my legs. She says, "We have a tube in there also. This is called a 'Catheter'. The tube has been inserted into your bladder so that you can pass urine during and after the operation. The Intensive Care Team can now measure how much urine your kidneys are producing."

The nurse looks at all the wires on my chest. She says, "You know what these are don't you?"

I half nod in agreement. She says, "These are called an ECG Monitor."

Now I know, I tell the nurse, "ECG, that stands for electrocardiogram."

"That's very good," says the nurse, "That's right."

The nurse sees my eyes drooping with weariness and tiredness. She says, "You are still feeling the effects of the anaesthetic wearing off. You shut your eyes and have a good sleep. It will do you a world of good," and I drift off into a deep restful sleep. I am awakened again by a bleeping sound. I look around myself. I see a whole host of electronic equipment still around me. I see the machine that's doing all the bleeping. It's this machine that's woken me up, it's going bleep, bleep, bleep. It must be monitoring my heart beat. Now I don't like to hear that. I see more monitors. They are all recording other important functions of my body. I see one monitor, it's recording my blood pressure by the looks of it. As I lay there in my bed I can feel my heart beating slow but strong now. I don't like to feel my heart beating. It agitates me. It always has done. I lay still and try to relax. The bleeping sound I hear, it's agitating me even more. All this is making my heart beat even stronger. Every time I feel my heart beat I can feel it shaking my chest. I can see the bleeping monitor by my bedside. It keeps on flashing a number up on its small display screen. When it first woke me up it was recording just below 80. It's now recording at 95.

I see a nurse come into my small ward. It's not the same nurse as when I went to sleep earlier. She's coming over to me. She's saying, "Whatever's the matter with you Doug?"

I tell her, "It's the bleeping machine that's agitating me."

She says, "Oh, that's nothing, it's only monitoring your heartbeat."

Them words from the nurse did it. My heart is now beating even faster. It's now racing on at a 102 beats a minute.

You readers who may be going in for a heart bypass must not be put off with what I am telling you. It's just me, I am an exception. I am squeamish to my heart beating. I always have been. The more I feel it beat the faster it does beat. The nurse tells me her name is Diane and that she is the night nurse and that she is looking after me. But Diane is in for a shock. She doesn't know about my past with my racing heartbeat. I never told anyone when I was admitted into the hospital for my bypass operation. Diane looks at the heart monitor. She says, "Don't pay any attention to the heart monitor, everything is fine. Just lay back and relax and try to go to sleep," and Diane goes off out of my small ward. I can see Diane sitting in her small nurses' room as I lay in my bed. She has full observation of me in my bed from her vantage position. I look at the hospital clock on the wall. It says 12 o'clock. I think to myself, is it 12 o'clock noon or is it 12 o'clock midnight. I can see the window from where I lay in my bed. It's pitch black outside there by the looks of it so it must be midnight and just coming into Tuesday morning. I try my best to relax as I lay in my bed but I can fair feel my heart thumping away. The bleeping heart monitor in my earhole is making things worse. It's making me even more aware of my pounding heart. It's going bleep, bleep, bleep in my earhole. I look up at the small display screen. I see my heart is now racing on at a 115 beats a minute.

Diane comes back to my bedside, she's saying, "Whatever's the matter with you, Doug?"

I tell Diane, "Look at the heart monitor." My heart, it's now racing on at a hundred and fifteen beats a minute.

Diane says, "I know, I have been watching the monitor in my room. You must try to relax and your heart will slow down It's a good healthy beat so don't worry. Now lay still and relax."

Diane goes back out of my ward and I see her go back and sit in her small nurses' room.

As I lay in my bed and try my best to relax I put my hand on my chest and gently tap to try to console my pounding heart. I feel something strange on my chest. I feel a strip of gauze or a bandage or something on my chest. I run my fingers up and down it. It runs from just below my neck right the way down my chest and to just below my ribcage. My left leg feels strange too. I reach down and have a feel. There's a length of gauze or bandage there too. I run my fingers along it. It goes from just below the top of my leg. It runs down the inside of my leg. I follow it with my fingers. It runs right down to just above my ankle. I don't feel any pain so I forget about what I have just felt. I lay back and try my best to relax. Just as Diane had told me to do. I can see the clock from where I lay. It's by now 2 o'clock in the morning. I can feel my heart. It's racing on more than ever by now It's fair pounding as I am trying to console it by tapping my hand gently on my chest. Diane comes back on to my ward. As she's coming to me she's saying, "Douglas you must relax. You're getting yourself all anxious."

Diane looks at the heart monitor. I look at the heart monitor. My heart, it's now racing on at a 125 beats a minute. I say to Diane anxiously, "Look at the heart monitor now."

Diane has seen the monitor alright. I will bet Diane has never seen a patient like me before, with a racing heartbeat like I have. I tell her, "This will test out the heart surgeon's surgical stitching" Diane nods in agreement.

It's by now getting late, late into the early morning. It's by now turned three o'clock as I look at the clock on the wall. I don't know if Diane gave me anything to sedate me, but she sat me up in bed so that I couldn't feel my heart beating and pounding as much. I must have drifted off to sleep. I now hear a voice calling, "Doug, Doug."

I open the slits of my eyes. There's someone looking at me as I lay in my bed. I think to myself, I know that face, it's Mr Munsch, my heart surgeon. He says he's been having a word with the night nurse, Diane.

"She tells me you have had a restless night after your bypass surgery."

Mr Munsch looks at the heart monitor by my bedside It's still bleep bleeping away to itself Mr Munsch says my heart has a nice healthy beat to it now. I tell Mr Munsch that my heart is usually a normal healthy beat, it's just that every now and again it goes haywire. It will beat and race on all day long, only slowing down to a nice healthy beat again once my body is physically and mentally exhausted of its energy. I tell Mr Munsch I have suffered a racing heart beat since I was early in my teens. I think it was the shotgun accident which I had when I shot myself in the wrist. I think it was the accident that made me squeamish at the sight of my own blood, even the blood suckers have difficulty taking a sample of my blood. I tell Mr Munsch all this goes back many, many years. It was not very long after I shot myself that's when my complaining began. I would go to see my old family doctor, which was Dr Palmer; everybody in my village knew Dr Palmer and Dr Palmer knew everybody in the village.

Dr Palmer would have me running on the spot in his surgery. Even in those distant days Dr Palmer would say, "You have a fine healthy heart there Doug."

Dr Palmer would comment and say, "I wish my heart was as healthy."

At that time Dr Palmer suffered with a bad heart and I tell Mr Munsch now, and here I am today still complaining about my racing heartbeat. Mr Munsch now tells me, now that I have had my heart bypass operation I will now feel my heart beating more prominently, "now that we have bypassed your blocked arteries your new bypass veins pass on the outside of your heart."

So I say to Mr Munsch, so it looks as though I am going to have a racing heartbeat for ever and ever. Mr Munsch says, "You have a fine healthy heartbeat there Doug, give me time to work on you and I will have your racing heartbeat sorted out in next to no time."

I wasn't to realise at that moment in time I will never be allowed to forget those wise shrewd words of Mr Munsch. I will come back to this part of the story a little later.

Mr Munsch tells me I have had a 'Double Heart Bypass' and not a Triple as first predicted. Mr Munsch carries on to say, "I have used a blood vessel from your chest for one of the grafts; it is called the internal mammary artery. The internal mammary artery is less likely to narrow over time than a vein graft. Mr Munsch continues on to say, "I have taken a blood vessel from your leg for the other graft."

Mr Munsch asks, "If I have any pain."

I tell him I can tell that someone has been inside my chest, but I have no pain whatsoever. Mr Munsch says, "Right, I have to go now. I am back on surgery shortly," and on that I bid Mr Munsch good day.

I look at the clock on the hospital wall. It says 7.30 am. I think to myself, these heart surgeons, they have plenty of work on their plates. Here it is only 7.30 in a morning and the heart surgeon is already at it. It was on the Tuesday, the day after my operation, that I was moved back onto the ward I was admitted into when I first arrived here at LGI. All the three same patients were still here who I had been introduced to earlier. I am laid on the top of my old original bed. I see a nurse come onto my ward. She's coming over to my bed. She says, "Right, Douglas. I am now going to change your dressings for you."

By the looks of it they need changing. Blood stained fluid had leaked onto my dressing. Now that my dressing is now removed I can now see the full extent of my scar. It's running the full length of my chest. I say to the nurse, "Where's all my stitches then."

The nurse says, "They have used internal dissolving stitches on you."

I see four longish lengths of surgical thread dangling there around the site of the chest drains. The nurse tells me, "These are tracer stitches. If complications now set in around your operation site, a quick pull on these tracers and you will be opened back up again instantly. As I lay there on top of my bed, while nurse tends to me, I feel something sharp sticking out at the base of my neck. The nurse says, "That's sharp wire you feel sticking our of your neck. Your Surgeon, Mr Munsch, has stitched up your ribcage by using a surgical wire and what you feel now is the end of the wire knot where it has been snipped off."

I say to nurse, "Will I have to endure this sharp wire now for the rest of my life."

The nurse answers my question. She says, "As time drifts on by, your body skin will grow over the prickly sharp wire and you won't even know it's there at all."

I tell nurse, "I have no pain."

"That's simply amazing."

I tell the nurse, "They can cut my ribcage wide open and I feel no pain. If I cut my finger it throbs and pulsates, but a big gaping wound I have got on my chest and I feel no pain. Incredible."

I tell nurse what Mr Munsch had told me earlier about him using my mammary artery from out of my chest. I say to nurse, "Now that the mammary artery has been taken away, how then does my blood supply get to it then."

Nurse answers my question.

"The left and right internal mammary arteries supply blood to the breastbones, but this area does also have other sources of blood supply."

Nurse now moves to tend the dressing on my leg. This leg is badly fluid stained also. I see big stitches here. They are strategically positioned along my leg. Nurse says, "The stitches in your leg are dissolving stitches and the one's you can see now will be taken out before you leave the hospital."

The nurse says, "Right Douglas, I am now going to sit you up in the armchair at the side of your bed."

As she says this the nurse has her back turned to me, so I gets up and sits myself in the armchair. I have upset nurse now. She tells me I could easily have exerted myself there and I should have waited for her assistance.

So here I am, now the Tuesday after my operation which was only yesterday, and I am now sitting out of my bed. As I sit there in my big armchair the sun's glaring on me as it shines through the window, I pull up a stool to rest my legs on and get myself laid back to catch a few rays of the old currant bun "Sun."

I am distracted as I lay there. There's Mr Munsch stood there. He has some of his fellow colleagues stood there with him.

"That's him," I hear them say.

"It doesn't look as though he's ever had an operation at all."

I open my chest front up to let the sun's rays put its healing powers onto my scarred hairless chest. As Mr Munsch and his colleagues are leaving my ward a nurse reappears. She says, "There's your clothes here Douglas."

"With what few clothes there is by the looks of them," I hear her mutter to herself. I ask the nurse, "Where has all my clothes been?"

Nurse says, "Don't worry. They have been in safe hands. We have had them in the overnight lock up while you had your operation."

As nurse is tucking a big pillow under my legs on top of my buffet, she says, "I make you comfortable Doug."

I look around my ward. I see all the other patients have their own personal television to their bed. Their TVs were all switched on. I look at my TV and its turned off. I ask nurse how I turn on my TV. Nurse tells me, "You have your own personal telephone at your bedside."

She gives me a number to ring. So I do as nurse bids and ring the number. A voice asks, "What network do I require?"

I tell them, "Television."

She asks, "Which hospital is that please?"

I tell her, "Leeds General Infirmary."

She now wants to know what ward I am on. When I tell her she says, "Oh, that's the cardiac ward, your television viewing is free. Hold on now, I am connecting you through."

She puts her 'phone down and on comes my television. I tell nurse who is still stood there, "My television viewing is free."

Nurse says, "It's funded by a donation charity for the cardiac wards."

And onto the screen comes one of my favourite sports programmes. It's a big snooker event that's taking place. This will keep me occupied while I am laid up in hospital. As I am laid back all fully absorbed watching the snooker, my ears prick up. I hear that familiar squeaking of a trolley wheel, and who should come in onto my ward but the nurse with the drugs and medicine trolley. She gives me tablets after tablets, all different shapes and sizes. She hands me two big white tablets. I say, "What do I do with these. Rub them on the top of my head?"

She tells me they are Paracetamols which are painkillers. She carries on to say, "Most patients after having such an operation as a heart bypass have got a scar down the length of their breastbone and a long scar down their leg, so the patients are bound to feel discomfort immediately after surgery, so this is what these Paracetamols are for; two to be taken four times a day and not rubbed on to the top of your head," and off nurse goes off out of the ward taking her squeaking trolley with her. My ears prick up, I hear squeaking trolley wheels clashing with squeaking trolley wheels. There's another squeaking trolley wheel coming onto my ward. It's the tea lady arriving with late evening tea, coffee, horlicks; whatever you want I am sure the tea lady is bound to have it. I order a large pot of strong Rosy Lee with not much use on the udder. The tea lass asks, "What's that in English?"

I tell the fair humble maiden, "It's a large cup of strong tea with not much milk in."

I now lay back on the top of my bed with my pot of Rosy Lee in hand and settle back to watch a late evening session of snooker.

As I am laid there my mind is half on the snooker and half on thinking of what Mr Munsch had told me only this morning. What was those wise words he said to me, I have a fine healthy heartbeat but I have to learn myself to relax and I can if I try hard enough to mentally train my heart to slow down. Now all this brought back distant memories I have, which relates to Mr Munsch's words.

I will tell you readers my story, then you will know as much as me as to what I am aiming to do. Many, many years ago now, I was on holiday in Spain. I see a placard up outside a theatre and what the placard said I like what I read. It was a show about a man who claims he can make some of his audience say and do anything he wishes them to. The showman was really a psychological worker of people's minds. The large theatre was full to capacity. The showman worked alone using the assistance of his audience all the time. He did quite a few tricks and the audience was gob smacked by his achievements. The showman had everybody sat on the edges of their seats. Now comes the part of the show I want to tell you the readers about.

The showman tells the audience this is his star part of the show, and that he will need assistance from people as he goes. He tells the audience what he intends to do. He is going to psychologically prime his mind, "NOT TO FEEL PAIN."

He is going to walk over a carpet of broken glass in his bare feet and when the jagged glass sticks into his feet, his feet will not bleed. To achieve this non-bleeding he must psychologically and mentally slow his heart down to nearly stop. That way the heart is not pumping blood around his body sufficiently enough to allow his feet to bleed. I think you readers might now have an idea why I wanted to tell you this showman's story. The showman beckons for assistance to come up onto the stage. He has big bags of glass bottles there. All the assistants now have a hammer, each have goggles on and protective clothing on. The showman leaves them to it to smash all the bottles up. The showman now beckons the audience and asks if there is a doctor in the house. No-one answers him. He asks then is there anyone in from the medical profession. A woman put up her hand. The showman beckons her up onto the stage. She tells the showman that she's a nurse from England. By now all the glass bottles have been smashed to smithereens. All the broken glass is now laid out in a long carpet like shape across the stage. The showman now invites people of the audience to come up onto the stage and check the broken jagged glass for themselves. Everyone agrees it is genuine and the edges of the glass have not been smoothed over. It's all sharp and pointed with razor sharp edges.

So the stage is now set for the showman's star performance. The showman goes back over to the waiting nurse who is stood by the stage microphone. The showman now sits himself down on a chair right by the side of the nurse. He rolls up his trouser bottoms, he takes off his shoes and socks. The nurse is asked to check the soles of his feet to see if there's no hidden protective skin over his feet. People come randomly from the audience to check out the showman's feet for themselves. Everyone is happy with what they see. They say they are truly unadulterated naked human feet. Everyone now is sat back quietly in the audience. Everyone sat on their tenterhooks, everyone totally transfixed on watching the showman. The showman still has the nurse by his side, he gives her a drum stick to hold. The showman is giving the nurse instructions. Us, in the audience, can hear her instructions as it comes over the microphone. She is stood again. When the showman's ready he is going to pass his arm over to the nurse who will take his pulse. Her instructions are to tap the showman's pulse rate out on the microphone with the drum stick. The showman tells the nurse he is now going to put his mind into a low psychological state of mind. He will practically stop breathing. He will put a polythene bag over his head and whatever the nurse may think she must not interfere with him.

"Just do as I have bid you."

The showman gets himself sat back in the chair. He passes his arm over to the nurse. She takes hold of the showman's wrist. She now has hold of his pulse. She starts tapping the microphone with the drum stick, keeping it to the rhythm of the showman's pulse rate. The nurse is tapping out a normal healthy pulse rate. The drum beats lessen rapidly. She's now got down to a tap pause tap and then the nurse stops tapping altogether. She's stood there with the drum stick over the microphone but she's nothing there to tap. With the nurse being a nurse, she's growing anxious as to what she is witnessing. The showman has no pulse. The nurse bends over him anxiously but she remembers the showman's strict orders. She must not interfere with him. All us in the audience, we are all sat there on the edges of our seats. We are all open mouthed and gob smacked. You could have heard a pin drop in the audience, it was silence everywhere around. The showman isn't dead after all. He pulls his arm away from the nurse. He takes his polythene bag from over his head. He's now stood up from his chair. He's now heading over towards the carpet of broken glass. You could tell just by looking at the showman he was now in a deep, deep physical and mental state. I am sure if the theatre had have been ablaze with fire, he wouldn't have known about it. He was in a complete world of his own.

The showman stops at the edge of the carpet of jagged glass. He ponders for a second. He now places his naked bare foot on the glass. He's now standing his full body weight on that foot, his face grimaces. He must be feeling some sort of pain as the glass must be sticking into the sole of his foot. The showman backs off the glass. There must be something there far too great for the showman to take. There's cameras situated along the carpet of glass so that us in the audience can get a close-up view of what's happening. The showman now stood back off the glass. The foot he had on the glass, he picks it up and pulls out a big pointed piece of glass that was stuck deep into the sole of his foot. By the looks of it he doesn't take kindly to pieces of glass that size. He throws it to one side. The showman again puts the same foot back on the carpet of glass, he again puts his full body weight on it. Glass can be heard crunching under his foot. The showman this time stands his ground. He now brings his other foot onto the scene and down on top of the glass goes this foot too. He slowly makes his way across the carpet of glass, feeling his feet down gingerly before setting his foot down. He makes his way to the far end of the carpet of glass and then steps off. There was silence from the audience. What the showman had just achieved deserved an outburst of applause. But the showman was in a deep, deep physical mental state. He asked us before hand to remain silent. The showman turns to face the carpet of glass yet again and off he sets again across the carpet of glass It's about 12 paces across and, oh, so slowly and carefully he reaches the end where he started. There's still no acknowledgement from the audience, we all remain silent.

The showman still in his deep, deep physical mental state, now slowly makes his way back to the nurse who is still stood by the microphone and still with her drum stick in her hand. The showman sits himself back down on his chair at the side of the nurse. There's a camera there also so that the audience can get a close-up view of what's happening. The showman picks up a foot and crosses it over his other leg. Big pieces of glass can be clearly seen stuck in the sole of his foot. The showman proceeds to pull out the glass that's embedded in his foot, and each piece he pulls out the camera clearly shows there's no blood. And, as the showman had told us all earlier, there's simply no blood because his heart isn't beating efficiently enough to circulate blood to his feet. The showman now lifts up his other foot and likewise does the same, and likewise there is no bleeding from the foot. The showman, now in a slow lethargic body movement sort of a way, he's still deep, deep and far away with himself. He puts on his socks and shoes and rolls back down his trouser bottoms.

The showman now sits back in his upright chair. He hands back his arm to the nurse. She quickly takes hold of his pulse. She's now poised with her drum stick over the microphone. She just stands there, but she's not tapping. The showman sits motionless, all us in the audience are sat there agog and in silence. Then we hear a tap, then a pause, then a tap and another tap, and then tap, tap, tap and the showman's heartbeat is beating all healthy again. The showman gets up onto his feet.

He's still looking a little groggy and dazed around his eyes, but he's okay. He's giving us all a bow from the stage. We all give him a big exploding applause. The vociferous shouting noisily of hand-clapping applauding was so noisy it nearly brought down the theatre roof onto the top of us.

So now you readers, I hope you all enjoyed my little story about the showman, and now you know exactly what I know of what I am about to tell you next. As I laid in my hospital bed half watching the snooker on the hospital's television my other half of my attention was being drawn away by the distant thoughts of the showman. I got myself to thinking, if that showman can slow his heart down to nearly stop, surely I can with some training slow my racing heartbeat down to a more slower healthier heartbeat. So, that night which was still only the day after my double heart bypass operation, Mr Munsch had also told me only a short while earlier, I could learn to slow my own heart down. I decided to give it a try. I turned off the television so that I had my own full concentration. I looked at the clock on the hospital wall. It was 11 o'clock at night. I closed my eyes, my heart was thumping hard but not racing on. If I could train it to stop thumping hard and make it beat at a more sedate beat, it would be a big achievement for me. I put my full concentration onto my thumping heart. The more I felt my heart thump, the more deeper concentration I put on my heart. I was forcibly stopping it thumping hard with my mind. I repeatedly kept attacking my heart with my deep thoughtful mind. I paused for a breather It's hard work is this deep mind over matter. As I lay there having a breather, I began to realise my heart now wasn't thumping as hard as it was. I was gaining control of my own heartbeat and at my first attempt. I needed more practice and training over my heart. I repeated again what I had just done earlier. After a little while, I had to stop and rest my mind. As I lay there, I couldn't believe what I was feeling. I couldn't feel my heart beating at all. My heart was completely and totally beating in slumber. That to me was a complete and miraculous achievement to me.

My mission now was being accomplished slowly but surely. It was by now 11.30 with the clock on the wall. I had gained a big achievement and all in the space of half an hour. I now took advantage of my slumbering heart and drifted off into a deep sleep. I will get back to this story a little bit later. I have much more to tell you.

Next thing, I hear someone saying, "Douglas."

I open one eye and have a look. I see a chocolate eye looking me in the eye. I open both eyes. I see a chocolate coloured lass. She has a great big smile on a chocolate coloured face. She says, "Douglas, what do you want for your breakfast."

She gives me time to wake up. She tells me she is called Dorcas. I comment she comes early with breakfast. I ask Dorcas what day is this? "Wednesday," says Dorcas. She has a menu in her hand. Dorcas tells me to choose what I want. There's a variety to choose from. I choose marmalade and bread and a glass of orange juice. I no sooner order than Dorcas has it there in front of me. Dorcas has another menu in her hand. She says, "If you order now, it will all be ready and waiting for you by midday."

As I am browsing the dinner menu, I am trying to get the butter out of the plastic small tub. When I look at it properly I see it's not butter but margarine. I tell Dorcas (she gives me that big chocolate face smile again). She says, "You're not allowed butter on this ward. Butter's bad for your heart."

The dinner time menu says choose your selected meal and tick the box at the side. So I did. The menu then said, now continue on and choose your selected dessert which I did, by ticking the box.

The menu then said, you will see a chocolate face lass walking around. You can't miss her. She's always smiling. They call her Dorcas. It says, now hand your menu to Dorcas and you will get your dinner prompt at midday. I think to myself, that menus nice and easy to follow and Dorcas doesn't take much finding. She's here laid on my bed. She's dropped my margarine down the back of my footboard on my bed.

Dorcas is now heading off out of my ward taking with her my now filled in menu.

After my breakfast I put my jeans and t-shirt on, slip on my slippers and get myself sat down in the big armchair by the side of my bed. The morning sunshine is fair powering through the hospital window. I have been writing a story for my book, so now is a good time for me to finish it. It's now nice and quiet on my ward. There's nobody to disturb me.

The story which I am writing about is a Lurcher bitch, which I once had. A Lurcher is a rough coated running dog. My Lurcher was called 'Gyp'. She was only small but what a crackerjack of a little bitch she was. She was my pride and joy. She was a sneak poacher. She learnt it all herself. I never ever learnt her, we would never go short of a rabbit, hare or pheasant for our dinner or a big fat farmyard cockerel, if the farmer wasn't looking. We would go short of nothing not while Gyp was around. So this story I was writing at my bedside that early morning in hospital.

Me and Gyp were going out early one morning to poach some rabbits. The woodland we were poaching was very heavily patrolled by gamekeepers, so me and Gyp had to be alert and have our wits about us. We were bolting rabbits out of the burrows with ferrets. Me and Gyp were that busy catching and killing rabbits when, as if from nowhere, the Gamekeeper jumped upon us. I set off to do a runner, I set off running across an open grass meadow. I look behind me. I also look over my bed as I am writing this story. I don't believe who I see. It's Gill. She's no doubt about it. Called to see how I am. Gill is a friend of mine. She lives in the same village as me. Gill is the secretary to Mr Nair, who is a heart surgeon at this hospital, the LGI. Gill will be thinking, I am passing close on by to Doug, so I will call in to see him. Just having my operation and all that, Gill may think I want cheering up. But that's anything but what I want. Gill has just come in right at the most important and exciting part of my story. I must not be broken off my story now. I must keep on writing. I reach into my locker as Gill is taking a seat by my side on my bed. I pull out a bag of bonfire toffee; it's that old style toffee where it's made in a big slab and then broken up into pieces. I look into the bag and pull out the biggest piece I could find. I give it to Gill. It was a real sticky piece. Gill's hesitating as she's looking at it in front of her nose. I can see Gill wants a helping hand with her big piece of sticky toffee. I stand up clumsily and on purpose I backhand Gill's hand that's holding her toffee. The toffee accidentally on purpose gets knocked into Gill's mouth. There I think the toffee is now where I want it. Gill is now reaching up to take it out of her mouth. I quickly look deep into Gill's eyes as I go to give her a kiss. Gill closes her eyes waiting for the unexpected. I put my hand under her jaw and push her jaw tight shut. The toffee is now doing its work. I pick up my writing pad. I see Gill out of the corner of my eye. She can't even get her finger in her mouth to dislodge the toffee. I leave her to it.

I am doing a runner across the open grass meadow, fleeing the pursuing Gamekeeper. When I am halfway across the meadow, I realise the gamekeeper's not in hot pursuit no more. I look behind me. I don't believe what I see. I see Gyp, she's running in and out and zigzagging between the gamekeeper's legs tripping him up as he's running. My faithful Gyp has come to my rescue. I take advantage and head to the safety of another woodland. Once there, I peep back through the hedgerow. The gamekeeper's now waving a big stick at her. The gamekeeper had a brace of pheasants on this stick. They have now gone. Gyp looks across the meadow. She sees I am clear. I see Gyp run behind the gamekeeper. She grabs into the grass and comes up with a brace of pheasant in her mouth. Gyp sets off for the safety of another woodland and away from me, luring the keeper after her with the keeper's pheasants in her mouth. I have learnt many tricks from Gyp. I know if I lay still Gyp will find me as I sit there waiting. I had to smile to myself with what I had just seen. I never learnt her to trip up gamekeepers, she learnt herself.

I see something bluey grey flashing through the woodland. It's Gyp. She's back. She comes over to me. She drops a brace of pheasants on my lap. That bitch was the apple of my eye in her heyday. I look up, Gill's making a move. She says she has to go now but "it's been nice seeing you up and well again."

I put my hand on to her cheek to give her a kiss. She backs off and says, "No, thank you."

As I am pleading clemency from Gill as she is leaving my ward, a little Chinese nurse comes in. She says, "Time for wash Douglas."

I say, "Oh that's okay, thank you, but I had a wash yesterday."

The Chinese nurse says, "You wash now."

She has me at my bedside, the curtain around us and has me all stripped off all within the flash of an eye. She tells me she is called, "Doris."

To me, Doris has a funny little titter, just like Frank Spencer in 'Some Mothers Do 'Ave 'Em'. Now Doris is taking my surgical dressing from my chest wound. In places it's stuck to my body with body leakage. Every time Doris pulls I give a wince, and every time I give a wince Doris pulls back and gives a Frank Spencer titter. It's taking Doris a long time to take off my dressing. Another nurse puts her head around the curtain. She says, "Haven't you got that dressing off yet Doris?"

Doris gives a little titter.

"It's stuck," she's saying. The nurse comes in and in one quick pull the dressing is now wrenched from my chest. Doris looks at me, I look at Doris. We both look at the nurse. The nurse says, "That's the way to do it Doris."

Doris now has a flannel all lathered up with soap. Doris is washing me oh so carefully around my chest wound. She's saying, "I don't want to get soap into the wound."

It's taking Doris ages to wash around my wound. The other nurse comes back. She has an ECG Monitor with her. She plays pop with Doris because she hasn't got me washed yet. The other nurse starts seeing to my leg while Doris is still on with my chest. The nurse has my leg dressing off in one quick pull. Doris gives a Frank Spencer titter as she hears the dressing zip and tear down my leg. She lathers Doris's flannel up with soap. Doris isn't using the flannel much anyway. The nurse has my leg washed and dried in a trice. The nurse says I now need a long surgical stocking on my leg to help the blood circulation. They are very close fitting, these stockings, so Doris and the nurse put it on between them. The nurse looks at Doris washing my chest, which is oh so careful, the nurse takes the flannel from Doris and gives my chest a good old scrub down with the soaped-up flannel. The nurse now leaves Doris to give me an ECG test. I am now alone with Doris. I am sure she can make a better job than Frank Spencer could.

Doris now has all the ECG wires out. She has many wires in her hand and many strewn across me. Doris has some wires under her feet. She bends down to unravel them. As she stands up she now has wires on top of her head. In walks the other nurse. Doris looked a picture as she's stood there with all the wires upon her. The nurse says, "Whatever are you doing Doris?"

She gives that quaint little Frank Spencer titter. Doris and the nurse wire me up together. The nurse has found a problem. Now she has put on my surgical stocking she now cannot put a wire onto my ankle. The nurse ponders the situation. She says, "We will have to roll the surgical stocking back down the leg."

I can see Doris thinking and using the powers of her wisdom. Doris tells the nurse her inspirations. Doris goes to my foot. There's a slit in the surgical stocking. Doris unfolds my foot through the slit and rolls the surgical stocking up above my ankle. Nurse compliments Doris on her astuteness, so Doris won the day. She was the worthy one to carry the nurse's trophy that day. Doris has now finished with me. Thank God for that. I think now for me to have a good old rest. I go to sit in my big chair by my bedside to catch a few old currant bun rays, 'Sun'. I bid Doris a little wave as she is leaving my ward. As Doris disappears another nurse now reappears. She's heading over to my bed. She says, "Douglas, I am going to get you walking a little around the ward."

So before I have time to sit down the nurse has me up on my feet again. She gets her arm locked through my arm and off we both toddle across my small ward. I walked with "aplomb", oh so easily, so the nurse leaves me to it, and to just walk around slowly on my ward. I wanted to go to the toilet. The nearest toilet to me was occupied so I go out of my ward and onto the hospital corridor. There's another toilet further along the corridor, so I head on up there. I have to agree with myself, this walking straight after surgery is really a bit of hard work. It was only Monday afternoon I had my heart bypass operation and it's now only about midday Wednesday and here I am trying to find my legs again. My legs were a little slow as I made my way along the hospital corridor. My chest also had a few creeks and groans and winces to it also, but I carried on going all in my own good time.

I reach my destination, the toilet. Inside there I see all the mod cons for the infirm patients. There's handrails for the toilet, handrails in the shower room, a specially designed lifting apparatus to get patients in and out of the bath. I am now finished. I now go back out onto the hospital corridor. There are many people about. There's doctors and nurses everywhere I look. Instead of heading back to my ward, I decide to head on the other way and further along up the long hospital corridor. All this steady walking will do me good. As I am slowly walking along there's other patients just like me walking the corridor getting the feelings of their legs again. Most have all had the same operation. Some are walking better than others; some are really struggling on with Zimmer frames and assisted by nurses. I bid each and everyone of them good day as we are passing each other by. I pass on by quite a number of small wards all just like my own small ward. I see patients in bed. Maybe they have just had their own operation. I see patients who have been got up out of bed and are now sitting in their big chairs by the side of their bed. As I reach the end of the long hospital corridor, there's another small ward. There's three or four patients I see are all sat by the sides of their beds. I see one patient sat there. He looks very familiar to me. He's reading a newspaper. I look closer. He's not reading the newspaper at all. He has the 'Playboy' magazine sandwiched between his newspaper. I move in and have a closer look. The chap has his back to me. I sneak a look at his face. I see it's my old friend, David. I pat him on the shoulder. David quickly closes up his newspaper. We are now re-united again. This is David I met a few weeks ago at teacher's classroom. I ask David where he bought the Playboy magazine from. I tell him I couldn't get one from the newspaper lass that comes around the hospital wards. David whispers, "Our lass, you know, Pauline. She's sneaked me it in. She says I have to be kept primed up through my operation, kept primed for 'bonking'. You know what Pauline's like."

David tells me he had his heart bypass operation two days before my operation. So on that, I shook David's hand and told him I will no doubt see him a bit later on, and off I go back down and along the long hospital corridor. All the patients I passed on the way up as they exercised their legs I am now passing them by back on my way down the long hospital corridor. As I am nearing my small ward I see a doctor in a white coat. I see him look at me. I hear him shout to a nurse, "Douglas Cox is here nurse."

I walk slowly into my ward. I hear behind me a squeaky trolley wheel. It's the nurse with the drugs medicine trolley. I tell the nurse I have been exercising my legs. The nurse says, "Yes, that's fine is that Douglas, but don't do too much too soon."

The nurse now hands me a whole host of different tablets I have to take. The nurse tells me to go have a good rest up now and while the day away. I have found just the right place to do this. There's a small lounge room, it's in between my small ward and another small ward. It's nice and cosy in there and reasonably quiet. There's just the odd nurse passes through the lounge to get to the other ward. I sit in the big plush chairs there in the lounge. I have a great big viewing window. With it being five storeys up I can see right across the top of Leeds city. There's a big tower clock outside, so I always have the time with me. I catch all the glorious sunshine that shines through the big window as I lay there in my big plush chair. I can see big aeroplanes flying low as they are coming into land and as they are taking off at nearby Leeds-Bradford Airport. As I lay there dozing with my feet up on the window ledges with the sun shining across my body, I will hear the nurses say as they are passing me by, "You look as though you're on your holidays Douglas," and also with the snooker tournament being on a free viewing hospital television I could lounge the evening away watching that, and I would drift off into oblivion and into a deep sleep. And, that's about all I can remember on that Wednesday I spent in the LG Infirmary after my double heart bypass operation. I woke up Thursday morning. My ward is busy already. I see Dorcas there with the breakfast trolley. I see the nurse there with the drugs medicine trolley and there's the newspaper lass with her trolley full of newspapers, and who's that I see coming onto my ward? She's sweeping the floor as she comes, it's my friend the sweeping lady. The newspaper lass comes across sporting all her wares to me. She says, "Newspapers, magazines, pop, Lucozade, sweets, crisps, biscuits," and do I want anything. I whisper in her pretty little ear, "It's the Playboy magazine I am wanting."

She shakes her head and says, "We don't have that sir."

Over comes the nurse with the drugs medicine trolley. Look at all the tablets she has there for me. They are like smarties all in there inside her small plastic tumbler. The nurse tells me to take them all now, they will make me a big strong boy. Over comes Dorcas with my breakfast of marmalade, margarine and bread and here comes the sweeper lady sweeping as she comes. Dorcas drops my marmalade, it rolls under my bed. The sweeper lady says, "I will get that."

With no fuss whatsoever she pushes her long handled brush under my bed and sweeps out my marmalade. Dorcas thanks the lady as she passes over the marmalade. I say to the cleaner lady, "My, that's a fine brush you have there in your hands."

The cleaner lady says, "Yes, this is the finest brush I have ever had. Just look at the width of the brush head. The dimensions of the brush head are far superior to other brushes I have had. It has a far larger sweeping capacity as I sweep."

Me and Dorcas are listening intently as the sweeper lady describes the workings of her new modified brush. The cleaner sweeper lady goes on to say, "Note the brush handle, it's fixed in a much more upright position. This eliminates having to bend the back all the time which, in turn, eliminates all stress on the spine and back muscles."

Me and Dorcas inspect the cleaner sweeper lady's brush. We say, "What a fine looking brush it is too."

The cleaner sweeper lady says, "It's quite unbelievable really. I have had this same brush now for seven long years and in all that time it's only needed six new brush heads and seven new brush handles and look at it now, it looks just like as new as the day I got it seven years ago. It's quite an unbelievable brush really," and off she goes sweeping the floor as she goes out of my ward and sweeping in an upright position. Dorcas now has my full attention. She says, "I have been telling my mam about you. I have told her that they call you Douglas. My mam says Douglas is a man's name to Dorcas."

I say, "So that means Dorcas is the woman's name to Douglas."

Dorcas says, "My mam wants to know what you do for a living."

I tell Dorcas I am a poacher.

"But," says Dorcas, "I thought poaching was only done hundreds of years ago, when poachers took the king's game."

I say to Dorcas, Well, they forgot to tell me poaching had finished."

Dorcas now wants me to fill in my menu for my dinner. I tell Dorcas that there isn't much fat on the meat here on the menu. Dorcas says, "You can't have fat to eat, not here on this ward you can't. Fat's bad for the heart."

Dorcas says, "There's a special dietician in charge of the cardiac heart wards, and they are very strict with the keeping a healthy diet on the menu."

I now have orders from the nurse. I am now allowed to take a shower, and I have orders that I must keep on leisurely exercising my legs. So I get my towel, soap, toothbrush and shaving tackle all together and off I leisurely go in search of a toilet with a shower. The nearest shower room to my ward is occupied. That's no problem. There's many toilets with showers to be found around these many small wards. I make my way leisurely along the hospital corridor. I can tell by the way I am walking. My legs are much improved on the day before's walking. I am not as stiff now. My legs are now more sure of themselves. My chest doesn't feel as tight and as heavy as the day before either. I am now passing by patients who I passed by the day before. They are out exercising their legs also. I bid them all greetings as we pass each other by. I come to a toilet with its door slightly ajar. I peer in, it's empty. I see a shower in there, so in I go. The hospital staff do not like you to lock the door behind you. That's so in case of any emergency they can now get into the toilet. I just close the door behind me and slot the little sign over which says 'ENGAGED'. That's about as private as I am going to get. So I now get myself stripped off and into the shower I step. I pull the waterproof shower curtain around myself and get myself wallowing under the nice temperature warm water. I let the warm water pitter-patter over my scarred chest. It's just like a warm massage as the warm shower spray of water soothes and cleanses my chest. I lift up my leg, I see the great long scar there. It's running down the full length of the inside of my leg. I give it the same soothing cleansing warm shower spray treatment as it massages my leg. While I now stand there just wallowing under the nice temperature shower spray, I let it massage my face as I clean my teeth. That job now done, out comes my shaving tackle. I never use a mirror to have a shave in. I always shave by touch. As the razor is passing over the thick hard stubble on my face, I can now feel with the sense of touch my face is now clean and smooth to my touch. A finer superior shave I acquire, I think, without using a mirror.

My shower now over, a quick rub down with the towel, and I now feel as fresh as a daisy. Once I am dressed all in fresh clean clothes which my sister brought me at visiting time on the ward, I now go back out onto the hospital corridor. I am still leisurely exercising my legs; the orders of the nurse. I head on further away from my ward and head on further up the hospital corridor. As I reach the top I look in on David's ward. I see Pauline there. She sees me, she comes over and gives me a big hug. I see in her bag a half hidden copy of a new Playboy magazine. I tell Pauline what David had told me earlier, "that you were keeping David sexually primed up with the Playboy magazines while he was getting over his operation. Pauline says, "Yes, that's right. It's my sex therapist who has advised me. She says the glamour girls in the Playboy will help to keep David sexually on the boil. This will help keep David all balls no brain."

I tell Pauline, "I can't get a Playboy magazine from the newspaper lass that comes around the hospital wards."

Pauline secretly ushers me one up my jumper. She says, "David's seen that Playboy."

I tell Pauline, "This Playboy you have given me is no good without a newspaper."

Pauline asks, "Why not?"

I tell Pauline, "I want to look at my Playboy magazine like David does, with the Playboy magazine sandwiched between the newspaper so then when I am looking at my Playboy the nurses that then pass me by, they will then think I am reading the newspaper, but in reality I am looking at the Playboy magazine. Pauline shakes her head in disbelief and gives me a newspaper. Pauline says, "What us women have to put up with to keep our man happy is unbelievable."

I now bid good day to David and Pauline and off I go with my Playboy magazine sandwiched between the newspaper and, yet again, when I arrive back at my ward, the nurse is again waiting to give me my tablets.

The nurse says I am looking nice and clean. I tell her, "I have been out on the corridor exercising my legs."

The nurse says, "Very good. You have worked well, you deserve a rest now. Go sit in your chair now by the side of your bed and have a read of your newspaper."

So that's just what I did, just like David, with my Playboy magazine sandwiched between my newspaper. As I sit there totally absorbed in looking at my Playboy-cum-newspaper absorbing the morning's sunshine as its strong rays are beaming through the window, I am disturbed by a nurse. She wants a sample of blood from me. As I close my newspaper around the Playboy, the nurse says, "Is there anything interesting to read in the newspaper today?"

I give the nurse a coy smile. As I sit there in a fear gripping sweat gripping minute while the nurse sucks my blood out of me, the nurse says, "Whatever's the matter with you Douglas?"

"It's the fear of seeing my own blood," I tell her. I catch a glimpse of my blood in her needle. I say, "Oh, it's the same colour as the blood I see on Casualty on television. I am sure one day I will get used to my blood being taken from me. There's nothing to it really.

In all the time throughout my stay here in the LGI, and after my double heart bypass operation, Mr Munsch, my heart surgeon, and his band of medical team have come to my bedside several times, forever and always wanting to keep up with my progress. Them asking me important questions and me asking my important questions. Mr Munsch's merry team of medical accomplices, they would often call to check on me and check all the medical notes at the end of my bed, looking at all the notes and reports that the nurses and doctors would leave in my confidential file. Nothing went by unobserved by Mr Munsch's medical team. I am now just about to get sat back down to read and look at my Playboy come newspaper, now that the blood sucking nurse has gone, when I see a porter come onto my ward. He has an empty wheelchair with him. He says, "Would you be Douglas Cox."

I give him a nod. He says, "Jump in here then, you're going for an x-ray."

So off we go. As we go along my part of the hospital corridor, I see someone has been putting up small Christmas trees, not too small I may add. There's decorative Christmas lights all lit up on the Christmas trees. They are bedecked with shining Christmas baubles. I like Christmas. I like the atmosphere it brings. I like its festiveness. I just like Christmas. As the porter pushes me along in my wheelchair we reach the top of my hospital corridor. I see another porter. He's coming out of David's ward. He has David sat in his wheelchair; he too is going for an x-ray. The porter drops in line with us and off we go along another hospital corridor. I see more people I know who have had heart bypass operations. These were all the people I met at teacher's classroom that day. They too were all in wheelchairs. They too were all going for an x-ray. They all dropped in line behind me and my porter. We come to the lifts; this is where I met them two dear old grannies that day, you know, the two grannies who didn't know if they wanted to go up or down in the lift. There were by now that many of us in wheelchairs we couldn't all get into one lift. Me and David were pushed into one lift and off we go. We get off at ground floor and we now reach a reception desk. It's a large reception area and the place is bedecked with Christmas trimmings and a big Christmas tree in the middle of the room. The tree was all lit up with Christmas lights and different coloured shining baubles. I see a decorative Christmas banner on the wall. It says, "MERRY CHRISTMAS 2005."

We are now booked in at the reception desk and off me and David go with our porters. David veers off to the right to some x-ray units there. I am taken a little further along and around another corner to more x-ray units. I go straight in for my x-ray. The porter says, "When I have my x-ray taken, wait here while I come back," and off the porter goes and leaves me. I have my x-ray taken in a trice. I am now waiting for my porter. I wait and wait until I get fed up of waiting. I remember nurses orders, "Keep on exercising your legs."

So I get up out of my wheelchair and have a saunter around the hospital corridors, admiring the Christmas decorations. I saunter on through the reception area. As I am near the lift someone presses the button for floor five. I think to myself that's where I want to be so I hop on. I get off at my floor. I now only have to go along the corridor a little way and I am back on my ward. I think, it will save my porter a lot of time if I get to my ward myself.

I am in no great hurry to get back to my ward so I just saunter along admiring the pictures on the walls of the corridor. I see some fine water colour paintings there. There's some, they look just like real life. The painters who do such masterful paintings such as these really captivate my eye. They are that realistic they are as good as if taken by camera. By the time I know it I am back on my own hospital corridor. I saunter on down and back into my small ward. The sunshine is still shining strongly through the window, so I get myself laid back in my big chair by the side of my bed. I stretch my legs out across the top of a buffet for a bit of extra comfort. I pick up my newspaper and start looking at my Playboy again. As I am sat there quiet, I see a nurse dash passed the entrance of my small ward. As she's dashing past I hear her say to someone, "Douglas Cox has gone missing down at the x-ray unit."

The nurse half looks into my ward as she's dashing past saying these words. A second or two passes by and the nurse backs herself back into view of my small ward entrance. She looks at me and dead in the eyes, she moves in closer. I start to shake. I see blood and snot coming down her nose. She says in a low blood curdling voice, "Do you know Douglas Cox, half the bloody hospital is looking for you."

She snatches my paper out of my hand. She says, "And you are all the time sat here reading this bloody newspaper."

As the nurse is saying this she looks at the newspaper, my Playboy is opened up at the middle page. There's a full coloured picture of the girl of the month. The nurse sees it. I look at the nurse. I don't like what I see. She looks to me as though she's trembling with fire and thunder inside herself. I tell her, "Calm down dear."

The nurse dashes off. She's wailing to herself, she's mourning out, "Where's Sister, where's Sister, she'll know what to do."

I think to myself, that nurse has lost it. She's flipped out. She's gone off her rocker and she's taken my Playboy with her.

The day passes uninterrupted. It's by now early evening. It's now dark outside so I go and sit in the lounge that's in between my ward and the next ward. I sit in there in the solitude and darkness not putting on the lights. It's best this way. I can now capture the atmosphere outside. As I sit there in my big plush armchair with my feet up on the window ledge, I look through my big viewing window; it's now different altogether outside there from how it looks in the daytime. I can now see all Leeds lit up. I can now see distant flashing lights high in the sky. As the flashing light gets closer and closer and lower and lower in the sky, I see it, it's nearly overhead now. It's a big massive aeroplane. It's that close I can see the pilot in the cockpit. I can see passengers looking out of the windows. They are dropping into Leeds Bradford Airport. I see another big massive aeroplane coming from behind me. It's climbing high into the sky. I see its flashing light getting smaller and smaller as it soars higher into the sky until it disappears into the darkness of the night. I see the clock tower. It's all lit up now. I check its time. As it chimes 6 o'clock (it's a minute fast by my watch) I hear the tea lady come with the early evening refreshments. She's on my small ward. I hear her shouting tea, coffee, Horlicks. I recognise that voice. I go into my small ward. I see its Dorcas; she tells me she's having to work late. I ask for a pot of strong Rosy Lee and easy on the udder Dorcas by now knows what that means. She brings me in a strong pot of tea with not much milk. I tell Dorcas to get one herself and come and sit with me in the lounge Dorcas tells me she's now finished for the day so she does as I ask.

As me and Dorcas are sat there snug in the dim of the lounge, Dorcas snuggles up to me. She says, "Tell me about your poaching."

I tell Dorcas about how I long net rabbits at night. I tell Dorcas I always poach alone. That way nobody knows nothing. I always start two hours after nightfall; that gives the rabbits plenty of time to get well out onto their feeding grounds. The night has to be black. When I hold my hand in front of my eyes I can just make out the lines on my hand. That's how dark it has to be. My eyes soon become accustomed to the darkness. I never use a lantern light. If I did the gamekeeper would see me and I don't want that do I? Dorcas shakes her head as she's listening to me intently. I take with me two long nets; each net is 100 yards long. I carry them in big large black sack. When the sack is draped over my shoulder the neck of the sack is tied at my waist. My hands must be free. I have to be prepared. The gamekeeper can pounce at any time There have been many bloody battles fought in the dead of the night in some lonely distant woodland.

I travel silently in the darkness of the gamekeeper's woodland. I get myself to where all the rabbits are. I sit at the side of a darkened woodland. This is where the large warrens are, where the rabbits lay up in the daytime. The rabbits now are feeding hard way out across the grass meadow in front of me. The wind will be hitting me hard in the face. The rabbits don't know I am there. The strong wind is blowing my scent away from them. As I sit there silently in the darkness up the woodland side I hear owls hooting and screeching at each other as they are talking to each other. They are saying in their own bird language, "Watch out, there's a stranger about."

They are talking about me. They have seen me with their big beady night eyes. The rabbits hear the owls also, but they don't understand owl language. I hear foxes barking and yapping at each other in some far off distant woodland. I peer my eyes through the darkness of the night. I see what I have been looking for. I see a distant lantern light in another woodland. That's the gamekeeper. He is out patrolling looking for me. His luck is out tonight. He is looking in the wrong place.

Dorcas huddles her arm tighter around my neck as she is listening, oh so intently.

It's now time to make my move and go in for the rabbit kill. As I get up from the woodland side I hear a scurry in the darkness of the woodland. It sounds like Billy, the badger by his grunting. He's only foraging the woodland for worms or the odd mouse or rat. Billy will do no harm to me unless he gets himself tangled in my net. I go silently and run out both my long nets up the woodland side. I have with me some knee length high wooden pegs. I silently push them into the ground and hang my long nets onto them. My now 200 yard length of nets are up and ready for the onslaught of rabbits. I have with me a great long length of nylon rope. I tie the rope to a tree at the woodland side. I now take a wide berth of the grass meadow where the rabbits are out feeding hard. My full length of rope is now outstretched across the meadow. The strong wind that is blowing is wafting my scent across the rabbits. My scent puts panic across all the rabbits. They bolt for the safety of their warrens in the woodland and they run headlong into my waiting nets I am still way out at the other side of the grass meadow. I hear rabbits screaming in the distance as the fleeing bolting rabbits ball themselves up in my nets. I lash and whip the rope across the meadow. There's rabbits still out here where I am. They are laid tight squat in the grass. A quick touch with my rope and they are up out of the grass and racing as if there's no tomorrow for the safety of the woodland. I hear more screaming rabbits as they are balling themselves up in the long nets.

I keep on lashing and whipping the rope as I drag it across the meadow. By now I am back at my nets up the dark woodland side. I see rabbits jumping and kicking in the net trying desperately to free themselves. Before I go in to kill them there will be more rabbits further down the nets. They will be sat just in front of my nets. They want a last final tup with my rope and they will all be safely in the nets.

That final job now done, I now go in to kill the rabbits with my thumb at the back of the neck and my fingers under his chin. A quick flick back of his head I hear and feel a slight click and the rabbit's neck is broken. I go down the full length of my nets in a frenzy of killing and leaving until I kill the last rabbit at the far end of my nets.

By now Dorcas is fair throttling me as she's gripping even harder around my neck. My knee feels wet. I think Dorcas has wet her knickers in all the excitement. My full length of nets are now full of dead rabbits. What a good kill I have had. Everything falls deadly silent. I now empty my nets of all the dead rabbits. I now pick up my nets and pop them back into their big black bag. I gather back in my long nylon rope. I gather all my rabbits together. There's a lonely narrow country lane not far away. With several trips I now have all my rabbits safely at the back of the hedge by the side of the country lane. I will gather these rabbits later with my Land Rover.

I now go back to the scene of the rabbit kill and pick up my gear. The night is only young. I head away and as I look back at the grass meadow which not long since was abounding with rabbits, there's not a trace of me ever being there at all. When the gamekeeper comes along all he will see is there are no rabbits there at all. I now continue on with my sack over my back. I am now heading for another distant lonely woodland. There are more rabbits there to be had. I will keep on long netting rabbits all night long, making sure I am off the gamekeeper's estate before daybreak, and that's the end of my poaching story I tell Dorcas.

Dorcas rushes off. She says she has to go to the toilet. By now it's getting late, late into the evening. I now go lay down on my bed. I watch a bit of late night snooker on the hospital television and drift off into a well earned sleep. And that's about all I can remember about that. Thursday I spent in the LGI after my double heart bypass operation. I am awakened next morning by people busying themselves on my ward. I see doctor's here, I see nurses there. There's cleaners and sweeper uppers. I see the breakfast lady, another lady I see. She has a trolley full of fresh water jugs. By now I have been at the LGI so long I have been acquainted with all the people that I know of them by their first names. It's by now Friday. It's by now going on four days since I had my double heart bypass operation. Surely by now I should be receiving orders soon that I am fit enough to go home. It's Christmas Eve tomorrow and I don't want to be in hospital for Christmas do I? I have walked my hospital corridor so many times now exercising my legs. I look behind me as I am walking. I see a groove I am leaving there; I have been up and down so many times.

As I am sat there in my armchair by the side of my bed sipping my Rosy Lee enjoying the early morning rays of sunshine, I see a nurse come onto my small ward. It's that same nurse that scarpered with my newspaper come Playboy magazine. She's coming over to my bed. She looks terribly revengeful in her face. All the blood and snot that was coming down her nose when she did a runner with my Playboy. It's now all gone. She must have had a wash since by the looks of it. She's coming across to my bedside with a determined look in her eyes. I don't like what I see. She has a pair of scissors in her hand. They are gleaming and sparkling in the sunshine that's shining through the window. She's now upon me. She pulls my curtain around my bed. She says in a rough agitated voice, "You, drop your britches."

With my britches half off she slumps herself onto my bedside. She's leaning all her weight across my body. I can't get up. She puts her hands into my groin. I think to myself, this is it, she's going to castrate me. I tell her, "Please don't, I was only looking at the pretty pictures in the Playboy magazine."

She's oblivious to all my pleads and plights. I hear the scissors snip as they cut. I feel a slight twinge of pain. I try to look over her shoulder to see what she's doing, but she pushes me back and I slump back onto my bed. I hear another snip of the scissors. I plead with her, "I don't deserve this."

She ignores my plights and keeps on snipping and cutting with her scissors. I feel her, she's now rubbing my leg. She gets up. She says, "There, all finished."

I look between my legs but I see no blood. I still look all intact by the looks of it. I now look at my leg, now I see what she's been doing. She's only been taking my stitches out of my leg. She tells me, "The rest of the stitches in my leg are internal stitches and will dissolve into my body."

I lay back on my bed and give out a big sigh of relief, as the nurse draws back my curtain. I am now bold and confident again. I ask her for my Playboy magazine back."

She says, "You can't have that back, Sister has confiscated it."

And off she disappears out of my small ward. As she walks out in walks another nurse. I recognise her face, it's my golden-haired angel who helped me through my heart bypass operation. It's Michelle. I tell her I haven't forgot her. She has a wheelchair with her. She tells me to hop in, we're going for a ride, so I hop and away we go.

As Michelle is pushing me along in the wheelchair along the long hospital corridors we go. Michelle tells me she is now going to assess my fitness on some flights of stairs. She says, "I know it will be especially difficult for you going up and down the stairs, but you must try your best. I think to myself, whatever is Michelle on about. I will have difficulty. Michelle now has me at the foot of her intended stairway where she is going to test out my fitness and ability to climb upstairs. Michelle pushes the wheelchair right to the foot of the first step. I get up quickly out of the wheelchair. Michelle hurries forwards to my assistance. She says, "Go steady Doug, you're going to fall."

So I stand there in front of the first step. Michelle's now bending down and holding my ankle. She lifts up my foot and places it on top of the first step. She's now easing up my body weight and onto my foot that's now on top of the first step. So Michelle now has me stood on top of the first step. I think to myself, whatever is Michelle doing. She's treating me like some shot up soldier who's just come off the front line in a war. She's now bending down again easing my foot up onto the second step. I lose my patience. I say, "Whatever's the matter with you woman. Let go of me."

I brush Michelle to one side and off I go up the first flight of stairs. Michelle races after me, but she's too slow. I reach the top of the first flight of stairs before her. Michelle is out of puff when she reaches me. She says, "Don't you ever do that again Doug. If you had fallen then I would have been in trouble with the hospital management."

There's now another flight of stairs Michelle wants me to go up and yet again Michele eases me to the foot of the first step. She's bending down yet again easing my foot onto the first step and yet again I lose my patience, and yet again I brush Michelle to one side and off I go up the flight of steps. Michelle was young and fit and carried no weight about her trim body, but she couldn't catch me going up that flight of stairs.

Michelle is puffed and out of breath when she reaches me at the top and yet again she plays holy hell with me. When Michelle has got her breath back, she says, "But you told me you would be no good at going up and down stairs."

I ask her, "When did I say that then?"

"In the operating theatre," says Michelle. I say, "Well, I don't remember ever telling you that, I must have been kidding you on. You're gullible to what I say Michelle."

Michelle says, I am gullible to what people tell me. I believe all they say."

I think to myself, so that's what Michelle meant as she was pushing me along the hospital corridors in the wheelchair. She was believing what I must have told her I would be no good going up and down stairs. Michelle has now got her breath back as we now both stand at the top of two flights of stairs.

Michelle now says, "I now want to see how you perform going down the stairs."

She puts my hand on the banister handrail. She's now stood in front of me ready to catch me in case I fall. She's now carefully easing my foot down onto the step below I am by now fed up with Michelle molly coddling me. I lose my patience with her yet again. I set off down the stairs brushing Michelle to one side as I pass her by. Michelle races off after me. She's shouting after me, "Stop Doug, you're going to hurt yourself."

I reach the bottom of the flight of stairs. I stand and wait for Michelle to catch up. Michelle's now upon me. She's just about to grab hold of me when I set off again down the next flight of steps. I race on and down I go. Michelle is in hysterics as she races after me. She's pleading and crying, "Please stop Doug, you're going to hurt yourself if you fall."

I reach the bottom of both flights of stairs well in front of Michelle. She's absolutely hysterical when she reaches me at the bottom. Michelle looks around to see if anyone had seen what's just gone off. There's no-one to be seen anywhere. Michelle ushers me back into the wheelchair. She gives me a clip around my earhole and off we both go along the hospital corridors with me in my wheelchair, every time I try to say something Michele keeps clipping me at the side of my earhole saying, "Shut up, you've done enough mischief for today, leaving me thinking Michelle's not the golden-haired angel I first thought she was. I get another clip around my earhole. Michelle says, "Stop thinking."

Later on that Friday afternoon, I am sitting in my armchair by the side of my bed when in walks Mr Munsch, my heart surgeon, followed by his team of merry colleagues and medical assistants. He tells me I have passed my fitness and ability test on the assessment stairway with flying colours and that I can now go home tomorrow, which is Saturday, the 24th of December, Christmas Eve. Mr Munsch asks about my racing heartbeat. I tell him since I had my heart bypass operation I have been trying with a lot of success to train my heart to slow down into a slumber. Mr Munsch is keen and all ears on what I tell him. He says, "Keep on training and learning; you have the ability to do just that."

And, in the meantime, he will determine the best tablets and medication for me to take, and working together we will settle down my heart. And, on that, Mr Munsch and his merry team of medical colleagues leave my small ward. And that's about all I can remember about that Friday after my double heart bypass operation.

Saturday finally arrives, it's Moving Day. I am eager and ready to be off home. I cast my mind back to what's gone off in the time I have spent here at Leeds General Infirmary. Come this afternoon it will be now five days since I had my double heart bypass operation. That simply amazes me. I have had my chest cut wide open, my heart surgically operated on, and then all stitched back up again, and here I am now, itching and ready to go home. All that major heart surgery and all within the short time of five short days. I feel "as fit as a butcher's dog, as strong as a bull. I feel that fit I could jump over the moon, and as happy as a pup with two tails."

All that has happened to me just simply amazes me.

My bags are now all packed and I am raring to be off home. Well, a quarter of a carrier bag full anyway. My sister, Ann, has been bringing me clean clothes everyday at visiting times and taking home my mucky clothes. That's why I haven't got much in my carrier bag. I now sit patiently waiting to go home. It's terribly stifling warm on my small ward. I see a window that opens. It wants opening to let a little fresh air in. It's just out of reach of me is the window so I pull up a chair to stand on. As I am trying to open the window which appears to be stuck, I hear a voice from behind me say, "You won't get out of there, so you might as well get down."

I look behind me. It's the Sister, it's that Sister which confiscated my Playboy magazine. She tells me to strip off to my waist and to lay on my bed. I dread what I see. She has a pair of sparkling shining scissors in her hand. The Sister now lays over me as I lay on my bed. She tells me she is going to take out the 'tracers' on my chest. I think that's what she called them anyway. As I told you before, these tracers are there for just in case anything goes wrong after my operation. A quick pull on these tracers and my whole chest opens up again. To look at the tracers, they look like two surgical stitches with four longish threads to them. They are situated just below my ribcage right at the bottom and at the end of where my surgical cut in my chest ends. As Sister is tending to my tracers, she says, "You are going home today."

Before I have time to answer her, I hear a quick snip and feel a sharp pull. I feel a strong twinge as I feel the tracer thread come from deep within my belly. Sister says, "It's okay, that was the worst one."

Sister says, "A passenger ambulance has been arranged to take you home some time later today," and all at the same time as Sister is speaking I hear another quick snip and feel another sharp pull. I feel another stronger twinge than before as I feel the tracer thread come from deeper within my belly. Sister says, "It's okay, it's all over now."

Sister is now getting up to leave. I pluck up courage and ask her for my Playboy magazine back. Sister says, "You can't have it back. I have confiscated it. I have taken it home to be disposed of properly."

Sister continues on to say, "When my husband saw the magazine he was alarmed at what he saw. He says he never knew there was such magazines about. He says leave the Playboy magazine with him and he will make sure it's disposed of properly," and off Sister goes and out of my small ward.

I am now aimlessly patiently waiting for the passenger ambulance to arrive to take me home. I ask a nurse when my ambulance is due to arrive for me. She says, "There's arrangements to be made first. We have to sort out all your medication tablets for you to take home with you. There is paperwork to be done also before you can go home."

So I wander about aimlessly patiently waiting. I see with it being Christmas Eve there are now many empty beds. Them patients that can go home for Christmas have gone home and them patients which are due for a heart bypass operation are now waiting for the Christmas period to be over. Usually, by what I have seen, all the beds are full, but now the only beds that are occupied are by those patients who cannot go home for Christmas. I see there aren't as many nurses and doctors around as per usual. It just looks like a skeleton staff that's on to me. It's by now well after midday and I am still patiently waiting for my ambulance to arrive. I know out here on the city streets of Leeds will be celebrating Christmas Eve. There's a pub I go in called the 'Three Legs'. I know by this time of the day that the pub will be full to capacity with people having a celebrating drink or two or three. I was itching to be in there with them. Just one celebrating glass of wine is all I ask for with my friends and fancy woman who I know will be in the Three Legs pub. It's only a 20 minutes walk away from where I am now in the LGI. I impatiently walk along the hospital corridor. I pass by Sister who is busying herself at her desk. I see her look at me. She can see I am eager to be off. I think she is thinking I am going to do a runner out of the hospital. She sends a nurse up to stand by the exit door. I go back to my small ward. There's a nurse there. She's been looking for me. I go sit down on my bed with her. She wants to know who I live with. I tell her I live with my sister and pup. The nurse says, "So that's two sisters you live with?"

I say, "No, just one sister, Pup is my dog."

The nurse says, "I have to check this out so that we know you will be looked after when you get home."

The nurse has with her tablets upon tablets. I say, "Are those tablets for everybody on my small ward?"

She says, "No, these tablets are all for you to take home."

She stuffs box after box of tablets into my carrier bag. She has a handful of leaflets in her hands. She says, "Take all these home and read them all carefully," and she pops them all into my quarter full carrier bag. It's not a quarter full now, it's stuffed tight with all her tablets she's stuffed in and all the leaflets. The nurse is now handing me a sealed envelope letter. She says, "Take this letter to your family doctor as soon as possible when you get home."

I say, "Is this a love letter from you to him."

She says, "No, it's all your private details telling your doctor what we have been doing for you while you have been in here at the LGI."

The nurse goes to put the letter into my now bulging carrier bag. She can't get the letter in so she says, "Here, put it into your pocket."

The nurse now leaves me sat on my bedside in my small ward.

By now I am fair itching to be off and, hopefully, to the Three Legs pub if I can. I saunter up and along the hospital corridor, oh so unassumingly. I pass on by Sister who is still busying herself at her desk. She looks over the top of her glasses at me. I see her look down the corridor. She gives the nurse the nod. The nurse moves to the exit door. I, oh so unconcerningly, turn around and go back to my small ward. The time by now is mid afternoon.

As I sit there on my small ward all fed up with myself, I have my head slumped down patiently impatiently waiting for my ambulance to arrive. I hear a chirpy happy little voice say, "Hi Doug."

I look up, I see my golden-haired angel, Michelle. She says, "She's called to pick up her signed book."

My sister had brought me a book only yesterday just for Michelle She's over the moon when she sees it. The front cover of my book has all be designed by me. It is a colourful cover all set in a nice shade of blue which is a picture all set in the wilds of the moorland hills with a picture of me leaning on a five barred gate watching a rabbit in a meadow in the foreground. Michelle wants me to sign her book to her son. As I am busying myself signing the book, in walks an ambulance driver onto my small ward. He has a wheelchair with him. He says, "Would you be Douglas Cox?"

"That I am," I tell him. He says, "Hop in, you're going home."

Michelle gives me a big hug and wishes me well, and just when I wasn't expecting it she gives me a big smacking kiss on my lips. I've now got to have another wash I tell her. I've had a wash already today. Michelle gives me a big broad smile that must have stretched from "ear to lug," as I leave my small ward. Wiping Michelle's lipstick from my lips as I was being pushed along in my wheelchair by the ambulance driver, we pass by the Sister who's still busying herself at her desk. I bid her a very Merry Christmas. She acknowledges me by looking over the top of her glasses and smiling. She tells the ambulance driver to keep on driving once he has me in the ambulance.

The driver says to me, "What's Sister mean by that then?"

We see the nurse who's still stood again the exit door. I bid her a very Merry Christmas. I see Sister give the nurse the nod. The nurse holds the door open for us to pass through. She says to the ambulance driver, "Keep on driving once he has me in the ambulance."

The driver says, "What's the nurse mean by that then?"

We carry on down through the hospital which brings us to the main entrance doors to Jubilee Wing and outside to the waiting parked up passenger ambulance. As the driver is bent down with his back to me while he is adjusting something to get my wheelchair in, I quickly jump out of the wheelchair and jump quickly into the passenger ambulance. I hate to be molly coddled. The driver turns to see me sat there in the ambulance. He has a quick look over his shoulders to see if anyone had seen what's just gone off. He quickly closes the ambulance door behind me, hops into the driver's seat and off we go. I look behind me as we are leaving and I quietly bid Jubilee Wing farewell, reminiscing the hilarious times I have had in there. It's by now coming in dark as we travel along in the ambulance. We travel along the headrow which is one of the main city streets of Leeds. I see Christmas lights bedecking the streets everywhere. It's just like a Christmas wonderland out there; the city streets are alive with last minute Christmas shoppers. It's just one big hustle and bustle of people.

We are now passing by my Three Legs pub. I look through the pub window and I see Little Joe. I recognise him by the back of his bald head. My eyes pop out when I see what I see. He has my fancy woman Sharon sat on his knee. Wait while I see Little Joe! It will be pistols drawn at dawn when I see him. I see Brenda the landlady, she's kicking out a drunk through the front door. I tell the ambulance driver to stop and drop me off here. There's Little Joe, he's pinching my fancy woman. The driver says he can't stop, it's more than his job is worth. We are now passing over Vicar Lane and onto Eastgate. These are another two main city streets of Leeds. We are now passing by Bolero Café where I often call to see Janet who caters there. The café is full to bursting with people. There's a party going off by the looks of it. I see Janet, she's shooting off party poppers. I shouldn't be here in this ambulance, I should be out there looking after my woman. I tell the driver he must stop, I must get out. He says, "I can't drop you off. I have been given orders to take you to a certain destination. If I drop you off here and you get injured, I will have to answer to my management. I leave all my sorrows behind me and we drive on. My village is Methley, only eight miles away. We soon arrive at my house. My sister, Ann, and Pup, my faithful bitch, come out to greet me home. I bid the driver a very Merry Christmas as he is leaving.

My house is a warm welcoming home. There's all the Christmas decorations up. The small Christmas tree is flashing with coloured lights. I settle down for a quiet evening in watching the television. Pup likes to watch the TV also. She's watching for the dogs coming on. On Saturday nights there's one of my favourite programmes on which is Casualty. I have seen them wiping up the blood in the emergency department and their blood is the same colour as my blood. Holby City is another of my favourite programmes. Mrs Beecham is a good surgeon. Connie they call her. She goes into the operating theatre and everybody jumps to attention; very upright is Connie.

The following day is Christmas Day. My sister is busy cooking the Christmas Dinner so I take Pup for a walk around the riverside to get a bit of fresh air into my lungs and build up an appetite for the Christmas Dinner. I come across a friend of mine. Les, they call him. Les has also had a heart bypass just like me but a long time earlier. We walk together along the riverside. We come to a bit of an incline. My legs and left hip ache but I carry on walking. I suppose it can be expected just coming out of hospital after major heart surgery and all that. Les confers with me about his symptoms he had when he first came out of hospital after his heart bypass operation. Les says he didn't come out of the house for the first month after his operation.

As the time and days went on by, I would walk around the fields and countryside with Pup. My calves in my legs and my left hip would ache. I would rest my legs a minute or two and then carry on walking, and my legs and hip would stop aching for quite a long distance before they would ache again. I would often bump into Les. He would say, "Is there two Dougie

Cox's. One that's fit and well and one that's had a double heart bypass."

I would shrug off my aching legs and hip and keep on walking.

Late January 2006, I get a letter. It's an appointment to see Mr Munsch, my heart surgeon at Leeds General Infirmary. The letter says I have to be there two hours before my appointment time. I have to have checks made on me beforehand. I have to have a blood test, a ECG and an x-ray, and please will I bring a urine sample with me. By now I am getting accustomed to going backwards and forwards to the Leeds General Infirmary. I take the public service bus as per usual to Leeds City Bus Station. I remember that bus journey very well. As I was getting off the bus, there was a fair maiden of a woman stood in front of me. As she was getting off the bus she steps down the large step to the pavement. She has a long skirt on that was near training the floor, so as she steps off the bus to my amazement her skirt comes clean off right in front of my very own eyes. She looks down at her dilemma She sees her lily white flowered knickers, just like I could see them. She gives out an embarrassed gasp. She looks at me, she looks at my feet. She sees my foot upon her skirt which now lays on the floor of the bus. She gives me a great big whack with her handbag right on the top of my head. She's now calling me all the names under the sun as she's trying to pull her skirt back on. Off she goes through the bus station with her skirt half on and half off. One side of her skirt was pulled right up still exposing her lily white flowered knickers. The other half of her skirt was trailing the ground tripping her up as she walked. She's looking back at me as she goes. She's still playing holy hell with me. I think she looks a little upset. Now she upsets me. When I look round I see my bus just leaving. Now, instead of walking the 40 minute journey to the hospital, I jump straight off my bus at Stand Six at the bus station and now jump straight onto the FREE city bus at Stand Three. There's usually a free city bus in the stand waiting. Everybody jumps onto the bus, no questions asked by the driver, no credentials, bus passes or tickets needed. At peak times of the day the bus is usually full to capacity. They are mini buses which seat around 30 people plus those who are standing. There are quite a number of these buses running which do a circular of Leeds city. All the buses run at staggered times, so you can see there's no waiting around for a bus to arrive.

So the bus is now full and off we all go. It leaves the bus station and off up Eastgate. If there's any room on the bus, the driver will stop to pick up more passengers or drop off passengers as we travel along. The bus turns left just before my pub, the Three Legs and on to Vicar Lane. We now travel along the main city streets and onto Leeds City Railway Station. Most of the people on the bus usually pile off here; they must all be catching a train. The bus is no sooner empty of its passengers when there's as many passengers getting on again. They must have all just got off a train in the railway station, so the bus is now full again with all new faces. The bus now leaves the railway station and on we all head around the main city streets. We pass on by the town hall where the four stone lions lay. Around the courthouses and magistrates court we go as we weave and turn around the city streets. The bus now stops as we pass near on by Leeds University. All the students on the bus all pile off here. The bus now sets off again a lot lighter of its passengers. We don't travel very far before it's my turn to get off the bus. I am now at Leeds General Infirmary . I have now saved myself a lot of walking. I now go into the main entrance on Jubilee Wing which is only just around the buildings from where the free city bus dropped me off.

As I stand in the main reception hall, I am looking for my appointment card letter. That now found, I am now fumbling about looking for my urine sample container. Here it is I have found it, it's stuck inside of my snotty handkerchief again. As I am looking down I hear a voice say, "Can I help you Sir?"

I look up. I know his face. It's that reception fellow who gave me directions before. He sees my face, he recognises me. I say to him, "No thank you. I don't want to go to the basement today."

As I set off to leave him, he takes his cap off to scratch his head, just like he did before. I now hop onto the lift and get off at the fifth floor, F Floor. I now know exactly where I am heading. No directions to be asked or required. I now know this part of the hospital like the back of my hand. I go straight to the reception desk and hand the receptionist my appointment card letter. She looks at the clock on the wall. She says, "That's good, you're two hours early for your appointment like we asked you."

The receptionist hands me back my appointment card letter now that she's booked me in as present. She's now sending me off to see the blood sucker. She's giving me directions on where to go. I tell her, "I know where the blood sucker's room is."

When I arrive there, there's nobody there sat waiting. The blood sucker's door is slightly open, so I put my head around the door. I see the blood sucker, she's laid back in a chair at her desk. She has her feet up with a cup of Rosy Lee in her hand. She's powdering her nose in her compact mirror. I say, "Douglas Cox reporting."

I startle her. She nearly drops her cup of Rosy Lee and her powder puff all at the same time. She says, "Fetch yourself in. I was just having a quick break in between patients."

The blood sucker draws my blood out with ease. I tell her, "Look, there's no sweating dripping fingers this time. My fears of you taking my blood have disappeared."

"That's very good," says blood sucker.

"Here, have one of the children's smarties."

She's now handing me back my appointment card letter. She's now sending me off to the ECG Department. She's now giving me directions on where to go. I tell her, "I know where the ECG Department is," and off I go.

When I arrive, there are many people sat there waiting for an ECG. The wooden holdall is still there on the wall. The notice on the wall at the side of the wooden holdall is still there, and it still says, "Please put all appointment card letters at the back."

By now I have grown all accustomed to all this. I look around. Everybody is that busy chin wagging and telling the tale, they haven't even noticed me stood there, so for a bit of devilment and to jump the queue, I put my appointment card letter at the front of all the appointment card letters in the wooden holdall. There's no-one even noticed I have put it there. As I am sitting down to wait (I know that's not for very long) the nurse comes out of her room. She picks up all the appointment card letters from out of the wooden holdall. She looks at the handful of letters in her hand. She shouts, "Douglas Cox," and off I go and follow the nurse into her room. I see all the waiting patients. They haven't even noticed what I have just done. They are still that busy chin wagging and telling the tale. They are none the wiser, as the nurse has me laid on her couch and wiring me all up. I say to her, "Make sure you put all the wire connections in the right places."

She says, "What makes you say that?"

I tell the nurse, "I will tell you a little story."

It happened way back in the 1980's. I was in hospital with something wrong with my left eye. As I lay in my hospital bed two nurses come onto my ward. They start wiring a chap up in a bed opposite me. The two nurses were doing an ECG test on him. One of the nurses looked a senior nurse by the looks of her uniform. As I lay in my bed I could hear them talking. The senior nurse kept giving instructions to the other nurse on where to position the ECG wires onto the patient's body. After they had done their ECG test I heard the patient ask if everything appeared okay. I hear the nurses say, "Yes, everything appears fine."

I see the nurses now move onto another patient in another bed and they do the same again and after they had carried out their ECG I hear that patient also ask, "Does everything appear okay?"

The two nurses' answer was, "Yes, everything appears fine?"

The two nurses now come to me in my bed. They want to do an ECG test on me. As the two nurses are wiring up my body, the senior nurse is called away to take a telephone call. The senior nurse says to the other nurse, "You carry on and complete the ECG test."

The nurse now carries on on her own. Her ECG test now completed the nurse has a serious concerning look on her face. I say, "Does everything appear okay."

The nurse says, "Oh, we don't tell you that."

Now, I do know they tell you that, I have just heard them telling the other two patients everything appeared okay with their ECG tests. Now I am growing concerned. The nurse dashes off out of my ward leaving me laid in my bed and still all wired up. The senior nurse comes dashing back onto my ward with the other nurse dashing on behind her. The senior nurse gives me the quick once-over. She soon finds the fault. The other nurse had put some of the ECG wires on in the wrong places. This had caused the ECG monitor to give out a wrong reading. The senior nurse quickly put the ECG wires in their right places and my ECG test is now carried out again. I ask again, "Does everything appear okay?"

The senior nurse says, "Yes, everything appears okay."

The senior nurse apologises to me for causing me alarm saying the other nurse is only learning. I ask the nurse at the LGI if she liked my little story of my ECG test I once had way back in the 1980's. The nurse acknowledges and says, "Well, us nurses, we are only human after all, and we do have to learn."

The nurse has by now completed my ECG test here at the LGI. I ask her, "Does everything appear okay."

She says with a big smile on her face, "Yes, everything appears fine. You look as strong as a bull to me, as fit as a butcher's dog."

My ECG wires now off, I am up and dressed and ready for off again.

The nurse now hands me back my appointment card letter. She's now sending me off for an x-ray. She's now giving me directions on where to go. I tell her, "That's okay. I know where the x-ray unit is."

I now head off from this Fourth Floor, E Floor, and down to B Floor, which is the bottom floor, or Ground Floor. This time I remember to hand in my appointment card letter in at the reception desk. I have no sooner handed my letter to the receptionist when a chap takes my letter from her. The chap looks at my letter. He's now shouting into the waiting room, "Douglas Cox."

I tug his jacket and say, "Here I am. I am Douglas Cox."

He says, "Follow me young man," and in no time at all I was in and out of the x-ray unit, all in a trice. The chap's now handing me back my appointment card letter. He's now sending me off back to the reception desk. He's telling me it's up on the Fourth Floor, E Floor. I tell him, "That's okay, I know where it is."

I remember it was at this moment in time I had to prove something to myself.

I know that before my heart bypass operation I went straight up these stairs here with no problems whatsoever. But, now with my aching legs and left hip I am not so sure of myself. I am now at the foot of the stairs, B Floor, which is Ground Floor. I set off up the stairs counting the steps as I go. I climb past C Floor, past D Floor, and up to E Floor. By now my legs and left hip are aching like hell. I have now climbed up 79 steps. I need to prove more to myself. I continue on up the stairs until I reach F Floor, 5th Floor. My legs and hip are aching more than ever. My legs feel like lead weights. That's 104 steps I have just climbed. I know before my heart bypass operation, which was only five weeks earlier, I had no problem climbing these stairs whatsoever. So I have now proved it to myself, something has happened to me since I have had my heart bypass operation. I now head back down the stairs to the floor below which is E Floor, 4th Floor and head onto the reception desk. I hand in my appointment card letter to the receptionist. She says, "By, you've been quick getting your tests done. I sent other patients well before you and they haven't arrived back yet."

She says, "Take a seat in the waiting room and your name will be called to see the heart surgeon. I take a seat at the side of an ornamental fish tank. As I am watching the exotic fish swimming around I see a notice chart on the wall. I go over and have a look at it. There's a picture of a heart. It's a diagram of heart bypass surgery. The notice says Atherosclerosis is narrowing of the arteries caused by fatty tissues. Atherosclerosis can also affect the hips and legs. These obstructions prevent enough blood from reaching your leg muscles as you exercise or walk. Without adequate blood flow the muscles are starved of oxygen and this causes pain. When you rest your muscles are not working as hard and require less blood flow so the pain goes away. For most people the condition in the legs will remain stable, or the symptoms will resolve with regular exercise and lifestyle changes.

Now, me having read this notice, I get myself to thinking, could I have atherosclerosis. The symptoms in my hip and legs are very similar to what this notice explains. I am distracted. I hear someone shout, "Douglas Cox."

I turn, I see a smart young chap stood there I acknowledge the chap and he beckons me into this Consultant's Room. As I am sat there at his desk with him, he tells me Mr Munsch, my heart surgeon, is not available to see me and that he is deputising for Mr Munsch. I look at the young chap's face I say to him, "I know you. I remember you from the LGI. You was one of Mr Munsch's team who helped me through my heart bypass operation."

The chap says, "Yes, I remember you too. It was you who didn't look as though you had had a heart bypass operation at all."

The young chap asks if I have any aches or pains in my chest. I tell him, "None whatsoever. I have never even had a single twinge of pain, even after my operation."

I remember I never told him about my aching hip and legs. This was all still new to me. I tell the chap, "The upper part of my left breast is still numb and the upper part of my shin bone above my ankle is numb also."

He tells me all this is due to my operation, and that it is still early days yet, and that over time the numbness should recover. The young chap is now checking over the results of all the tests I have just had here today. He comments on my cholesterol. He says, "It was sky high at 8.5 when you had your heart attack in September 2005, but I see it's fine now at a healthy 4.2."

The chap's now looking at my blood test results. He says, "That's fine."

My ECG is fine, my urine test is fine. He's now holding up to the light my x-ray photo. He says, "That's fine also."

The young chap gets up from his seat. He shakes my hand. He says, "There, I don't want to see you no more. You are now all fit and well again. You can now carry on and do as you've always done, but take a more leisurely approach," and on that he now says, "I am now discharging you after only five short weeks."

On that I bid the young chap good day and off I went home. The notice board chart I have just read in the reception area, the word atheroslcerosis, keeps ringing in my ears. The symptoms, it explains, are very near the symptoms I have in my legs and left hip, but I am convinced my symptoms came on to me far too quick for it to be atherosclerosis. There's something that has happened to me since I had my double heart bypass operation. In my mind there's only one thing that can be making my legs and hip ache and that's the heart tablets I am taking.

So not long after, I go to see my family doctor. Mrs Dunphy, they call her. A really nice woman is Mrs Dunphy. I know that because she's always telling me she's a really nice woman but, for some reason, I always seem to stretch her patience. Over the time since my operation, I have been to see Mrs Dunphy on several occasions. She likes to keep me in check and underhand, always checking my blood pressure and cholesterol level, and each time I have seen her I have told her about my aching legs and left hip. As I sit in the doctor's waiting room I hear my name being called over the tannoy system, "Douglas Cox" Room One please."

It sounds like a shaky voice from Mrs Dunphy. She beckons me in as I knock on the surgery door. She has her back to me as I go in. She says, "Would you like a drink of tea?"

I say, "I wouldn't mind a cup of Rosy Lee."

As I sit myself down, Mrs Dunphy has nowhere to put my cup of Rosy Lee, so I rearrange her desk for her and push everything over a little. There I can now get my elbow on her desk. Mrs Dunphy sits herself down and pushes everything back across her desk, back to where it all was in the first place. Mrs Dunphy asks how I went on with my recent appointment at the LGI. I tell her I have now been discharged after only five short weeks. I tell her about the notice board on which I read all about atherosclerosis. Mrs Dunphy says, "It could be that which is giving you poor blood circulation to your legs and hip. It could also be the medication tablets that you are taking," says Mrs Dunphy. I say, "It's got to be the tablets. I am told that walking is good for my heart, but it's the tablets that are causing my legs to ache which makes me less interested in walking."

I see Mrs Dunphy go deep into thought. I push her blood pressure arm band tester across her desk. There, I can get my elbow on the desk again. Mrs Dunphy is now looking at her computer.

"I see here," says Mrs Dunphy, "that your cholesterol was high at 8.2 back in September and that the 40mg Simvastatin tablets brought your cholesterol down to a healthy 4.2, and the tablets that you are on now are Simvastatin, Bisoprolol, Perindopril and Aspirin."

Mrs Dunphy looks up from her computer. She pushes her blood pressure arm band tester back to where it was on her desk. Mrs Dunphy is becoming agitated. She tells me to leave her blood pressure tester alone and to leave everything else alone on her desk also.

Mrs Dunphy says, "What I am going to do is a process of elimination of all the tablets you are taking. We will eliminate the tablets one at a time to see if it's the tablets that are making your legs and hip ache. We can eliminate the aspirin straight away. It will not be them I am sure," says Mrs Dunphy.

"Firstly, we shall eliminate the 40mg Simvastatin. I will put you on an alternative tablet called Salvastatin which will also keep your cholesterol in check. The process of elimination of the Simvastatin will be over a six week period."

Mrs Dunphy gets up from her seat. She asks, "Would I like another cup of Rosy Lee?"

She says in an agitated voice, "Look, you've got me calling it Rosy Lee now."

While Mrs Dunphy has got her back turned to me, while she's making the Rosy Lee, I think to myself Mrs Dunphy said earlier my cholesterol was high at 8.2 back in September 2005. Her computer must be wrong. My cholesterol was 8.5 back in September 2005, so while Mrs Dunphy has her back turned on me I push her blood pressure tester back across her desk. I swivel her computer around to check on my cholesterol myself. She has the computer turned on at the wrong page, so I press a button to alter the page. Everything on the screen goes blank. I press another button and another page goes blank. Mrs Dunphy turns around with a cup of Rosy Lee in each hand. She sees the blank computer screen. She's up in arms at what she sees. I look at her. I don't like what I see. She looks all confused and confounded. She pulls her computer out of my grasp. She sees I have moved her blood pressure tester again. She slams it back to where it was again. As she slams it she knocks a tray full of doctors' documents which fall from her desk and scatter all over the surgery floor. Mrs Dunphy now has her hands over her face. She's peeping through her fingers. I am now sure I don't like what I see. I am now heading for the door. I tell Mrs Dunphy I haven't got time to drink her Rosy Lee and I will be back to see her in six weeks' time. She's always getting herself upset with me is Mrs Dunphy. I don't know why. As I am heading past the reception area I see my friend David. He's trying to work the computer on the wall. He asks me how it works.

This computer on the wall is new day technology. So now, instead of letting the receptionist know of your arrival for your doctor's appointment, you just simply press a few buttons on the computer on the wall and it books you all in that you have arrived. So, as I am showing David how the computer works we hear a hysterical woman mourning out. It's Mrs Dunphy. She's telling the receptionist ladies. She's pulling and tearing at her hair, she's mourning out, "It's that Douglas Cox, he's erased all my medical information on my computer. All my medical documents are strewn all over the surgery floor."

Mrs Dunphy looks across, she sees me. She mourns out hysterically. She's pointing a finger at me. In a pitiful state of mind she says, "That's him," repeatedly saying, "That's him."

David says, "This computer, the screen's gone all blank."

I leave everybody to it and off I go.

Over the six weeks' trial period I walked the fields and countryside with Pup, my faithful bitch. I was still fit enough and able enough to outpace the gamekeeper when he came upon us poaching his rabbits. It takes about six weeks for the drug, Simvastatin, to wear out of my system. After five weeks of trialling I had to go back to my family doctors. Mrs Dunphy wanted me blood tested. She was keeping a close eye on my cholesterol level. The following week I had to go to see Mrs Dunphy at our local village surgery. As I go to the computer on the wall to book myself in as arrived and present the receptionist sees me and comes dashing from around her reception room. She says, "I will book you in Doug, it will save getting out the computer electrician."

As I sit in the doctors' waiting room I hear over the tannoy system an uneasy voice of Mrs Dunphy, "Douglas Cox, Room One please."

Mrs Dunphy beckons me in as I knock on her surgery door. I see Mrs Dunphy has moved her computer. I see that everything else on her desk has been moved also. I take a seat while Mrs Dunphy is looking on her computer. She says, "Your blood test results have arrived back and your cholesterol level has gone up from 4.2 to 5.2. The Salvastatin tablets are not keeping your cholesterol down as well as the Simvastatin tablets, so I will have to put you back on the 40mg Simvastatin tablets."

I say, "That's just as well, the six weeks trial of the tablets have not been a success. My legs and left hip still ache after I have walked a fair distance."

Mrs Dunphy says, "And your legs and hip do not ache when you are at rests?"

I say, "No, only when I walk a fair distance."

Over the following 12 weeks, I trialled the other two tablets I was taking, not taking the Perindopril tablets for a six week period. That was a failure; my legs and left hip still ached while walking a fair distance. I then trialled the Bisoprolol tablets for another further six weeks period which was also a failure and my legs and left hip would ache only when I walked a fair distance. So now Mrs Dunphy's trial of all the tablets I was taking was now over. Mrs Dunphy now says, "I am now going to send you off to hospital to get your legs checked out to see if it's poor blood circulation that's affecting your legs and making them ache."

Mrs Dunphy sends me off to see her secretary. Mrs Dunphy's secretary is only next door and she sees me straight away. She tells me it's a new system they have now for booking an appointment at the hospital. She tells me I can choose any hospital I wish to attend in my local vast area which has many hospitals. I select Pinderfields Hospital which is convenient for me. The secretary is now handing me a letter. She says, "You, yourself, book your own appointment."

She points to a telephone number on my letter she has just given me, saying, "That's the headquarters for all the district hospitals."

I telephone for an appointment from my home. I ring the telephone number on my letter and I get straight through. I inform them what I require. I have a PIN reference number on my letter which I tell them, and that's all there was to it. They tell me I will be receiving my appointment date through the post, so all I have to do now is wait for my appointment to arrive.

By now it's the month of late March 2006. A letter drops through my letterbox. I see it's an appointment for an outpatients visit to Pinderfields Hospital at Wakefield. But its not the appointment I have been waiting for to have my aching legs and hip checked out, it's an appointment for me to see Mr Phil Batin, the Cardiologist. This is the chap who diagnosed my heart condition on the angiogram machine when I was rushed into Pinderfields Hospital with my heart attack way back in September 2005. The letter says this is an important appointment for me to see Mr Phil Batin, the Heart Specialist. It will allow the doctors to assess how well you are recovering and give them the chance to change your medicines if necessary. They also give you the chance to ask any questions or ask about any symptoms you have had during your recovery period and which may be troubling you. Before you go for your appointment, you may find it helpful to write down any questions you want to ask the doctor. If you do not understand something the doctor says it's okay to ask him to explain it to you again, or in a different way. Before the end of your appointment make sure that they have answered all your questions. It says at the bottom of the letter, PS If you do not receive this letter please inform the above address.

So off I go to my appointment. As I sit in the waiting room I hear my name called. I turn, I see, I recognise that face from the past. It's Mr Phil Batin, my Cardiologist, 'heart surgeon'. I follow him into his consulting room. He shakes my hand just like a true English gentleman. Mr Batin comments that I am looking very fit and well. He asks if I have any aches or pains in my chest. I tell him, "None whatsoever, not even after my operation when they cut my chest wide open."

He's now checking all the tablets I am taking.

"They look fine," says Mr Batin. He now asks if I have any numbness in my chest or leg. I tell him that I have. He asks me to explain the numbness. I tell him, "The upper part of my left breast is numb to the touch."

Mr Batin says, "That's to be expected. Mr Munsch who operated on your heart did take your mammary blood vessel from your left breast, but the numbness in your breast will recover over time, and the numbness in your left leg," says Mr Batin. I tell him, "The numbness is just above my ankle on the inside of my shin bone."

Mr Batin's reply was, "During your heart bypass operation Mr Munsch took the blood vessel from the full length of your leg and the numbness you have was to be expected. Mr Batin sees me touching the bottom of my throat just above my chest. He asks if the prickly wire has disappeared yet."

I tell him, "Yes, it has."

He explains, "After your operation Mr Munsch stitched your ribcage back together with surgical wire for strength. When he tied off the wire which is at the top or your chest now where you are touching, once he has snipped off the surplus wire it leaves a prickly bit sticking out, but time sorts it out. Just like it has done with you, the body skin grows over the protruding wire and covers it over."

I now seize the chance and ask Mr Batin about my aching legs and left hip. I tell him, "They did not ache before my heart bypass operation."

Mr Batin answered my question without even pondering. He says, "It's the heart tablets that you are taking."

He asks if I have any more questions for him. I say, "Yes, I have another question for you. Now that my big long blood vessel has been removed from the full length of my left leg, how does my blood circulation get down to my foot and back up my leg again?"

Mr Batin smiles and says, "Good question Doug."

He explains, "If you are driving your car outside on the main Aberford-Wakefield road (as he points to the main road that runs past Pinderfields Hospital), if that road blocked up with a traffic jam, you wouldn't just sit there would you? You would find alternative side roads to get you by the traffic jam wouldn't you?"

I nod in agreement. Mr Batin continues to say, "Your blood circulation in your legs is just the same. Your blood finds an alternative route. There are many small blood vessels in your leg for your blood to follow."

So, that answered my question in straight 'John Bull layman's terms'.

There's something nattering my mind. I don't think Mr Batin answered my question clearly enough when he said it was the tablets that was causing my legs and hip to ache, so I ask Mr Batin again. He says, "The tablets affect some people more than others. Your aching legs and hip may resolve themselves with exercise and a lot of walking just like you do Doug on the fields. Getting chased by the gamekeeper now and then will do your legs good also."

So the answer Mr Batin gave me was what that notice chart told me when I saw it on the wall recently at Leeds General Infirmary. Mr Batin says, "I am now discharging you. You are now fit and well. Carry on your life as per normal but take things at a more leisurely pace. All you have to do now is go for an ECG which has all been arranged for you. After your ECG you can then go home. I don't want to see you no more."

And on that I shook hands with Mr Batin and bid him good day.

So, after three short months, after having my double heart bypass operation, I am now discharged from hospital altogether. After having my ECG done by the nurse, I get myself ready for home. The nurse says, "You can't go home yet, Mr Batin needs to see the ECG results first."

I tell the nurse, "Mr Batin has told me, when I have had my ECG I can go straight home after."

The nurse says, "I will go check with Mr Batin."

The nurse is not long before she's back. She says, "Yes, you can now go home. Mr Batin must have some sort of supernatural powers. He says you're fit and well enough to go home. How's he know that without seeing your ECG results," says the nurse, and on that off I go homeward bound. Not very long after this appointment I have just had with Mr Batin, another letter drops through my letterbox. It's the appointment I have been waiting for. It's to have my aching legs and hip checked out. It's at the same place, Pinderfields Hospital, Wakefield. So off I go to meet my appointment.

When I arrive at the main reception desk the receptionist looks at my letter. There's a big tall chap stood again us. She beckons him over. The receptionist tells the chap where I want to be. The chap says, "Follow me young man," and off the chap sets striding out at a fair pace. We go along the long hospital corridors, turning this way and that way. The tall chap doesn't know I have just had a double heart bypass. He doesn't know my legs and hip ache with walking a fair distance, but as he paces out along the long hospital corridors I am adamant I am going to keep up with him. I say to the tall chap, "You must walk a fair distance in a week walking all these rabbit warren hospital corridors."

"Not really," he says, "I am a voluntary worker, guiding patients to their destinations. I only do it Thursday mornings."

We eventually come to a stop. We are by now right at the other side of the hospital. The tall chap points from a doorway to another doorway across the block. He says, "That's where I want to be."

I head across to the block and onto the reception desk. There are many patients there in the waiting room. It looks like some sort of casualty department to me. There appears to be a lot of walking wounded around. There's a chap there with all his head bandaged up. I see another with his arm in a sling. There's another chap at the back of me in the receptionist's queue. He keeps on knocking into me as I stand there. I see he's unstable on a pair of crutches. There's a commotion over by the entrance door. I see another walking wounded coming in. He's being helped in by another chap. It's the casualty's mate by the looks of it. They both push themselves to the front of the queue in front of me. The casualty tells the receptionist in a slurred drunken manner, "I have been in a fighting brawl."

His face is all covered in blood, his front teeth have been kicked in. I see his nose is bent to one side. It looks broken to me. The receptionist says to the drunken casualty as she's looking at his blood covered face, "Right, can you tell me where you have been injured."

The blood covered casualty slurs out to the receptionist, "Are you trying to be funny? Do you need some specs or what?"

The receptionist hands him a doctor's introductory referral note to be passed onto the casualty doctor. She says, "Here, take this and go sit down in the waiting room."

The drunken casualty takes the note from her. He screws it up into a ball and puts it into his mouth and starts chewing it up. The receptionist looks gob smacked at seeing what she's just seen. She says to me, "There, I have seen it all now."

As the drunken casualty is walking away I hear him say to his mate, "There, I feel a lot better now I have taken that."

The receptionist now deals with me and I go and sit down in the waiting room.

I sit myself down at the side of the drunken casualty. I say to him, "By, you've had a drop of good ale down you by the looks of you."

I ask him which pub he has been in. He says with a drunken slurred up tongue, "It's in Wakefield Town Centre, they call the pub 'A Man in a Trance'."

Now, that got me scratching my head. There's no pub called that in the town centre. I remember when I had finished at this hospital that day, I went to that place where the drunken casualty had told me where the pub was. It read over the pub door in big letters, 'MAIN ENTRANCE'. I suppose it reads like that to a drunken man.

As I sit there I see another chap come in. He sees the chap next to me. He knows him. These are the words I hear them speak, "Now then Harry, how are you going on?"

Harry says, "I am not too clever Eric. I am constipated. I am all bunged up. I can't shit."

Eric says, "All you want is some suppositories. They will make you shit through the eye of a needle."

Harry says, "I have taken suppositories after suppositories until I am fed up of taking suppositories. For what good they have done me I might as well have pushed them up my arse."

As I sit there in the waiting room patiently waiting for my name to be called, I see another chap come in. I know his face. It's my friend, David. He comes over and sits down by my side. I see he has a pot on his foot. David tells me he broke his ankle and has come to have his pot removed. David's not sat there for long before the nurse shouts him into her nurses' room. David leaves the door slightly open. I can see right into the nurses' room which is at the side of me where I am sitting. I see the nurse take off David's plaster cast. I hear the nurse say to David, "Now, just walk up and down and let me see that it hasn't left you with a limp. So David walks up the room and back again. I see the nurse use her professional astuteness. She says to David, "It's left you with a limp."

Now, David has a stuttering, stammering voice. He says to the nurse in a stuttering voice "It hasn't left me with a limp. I am limping because I have my shoe on my other foot."

Again, the nurse uses her astute shrewdness. She says, "No, it's not because of your shoe."

David says in an excited stuttering, stammering voice, "Look I will show you."

David takes off his other shoe. His big toe is stuck out from a hole in his sock. He now walks along the room and back again. David says, "There, I am not limping now am I."

The nurse agrees David is not now limping. I am distracted. I hear my name being called. I see a nurse, I acknowledge her. She beckons me to follow her, and off we go and into her nurses' room.

As we sit there she introduces herself as Sonia. Sonia reads my personal medical notes. She sees that I want my aching legs and hip checking out. Firstly, Sonia wants to check out my lifestyle. She asks what my occupation is. I tell Sonia, "Poacher."

That amuses Sonia. She says, "I have heard many a patient's occupation over my time, but poacher beats the lot of them."

I tell Sonia, "It was my lifestyle being brought up as a poacher, but over the last 25 years I have been a full-time rabbit catcher for the Lords of the Manor, getting the finest of the fresh air in the hilltops up in the Yorkshire Dales. I tell Sonia, "I have written a book all about my lifestyle."

Sonia appears impressed at what I tell her and agrees I have led a healthy lifestyle. Sonia now looks at the tablet medications I am taking. I tell Sonia about my family doctor, Mrs Dunphy and how we did the process of elimination of each of the tablets to see if it was any of the individual tablets that was making my legs and left hip ache.

"What were the results?"

asks Sonia.

"A failure," I say. Sonia beckons me onto her couch and tells me to take off my britches. Sonia's now smearing jelly on certain points on my legs and hips. She now has some sort of handset in her hand. She's now putting the handset onto the inside of my groin. I hear amplified pulsating sounds as my heart pumped blood through my legs. I ask Sonia what it sounds like. She says, "Your blood circulation is fine there."

Sonia now moves her handset to around my knee. Again I hear amplified pulsating sounds. Again, I ask Sonia the same question and again Sonia says, "Your blood circulation is fine there also."

Sonia's now moving her handset to around my ankle, and Sonia says again, "Your blood circulation if fine there also."

Sonia does exactly the same on my other leg and says, "The blood circulation is fine on that leg also."

So I say, "So that's all good news."

Sonia nods in agreement. Sonia tells me to put on my britches and go sit back at her desk. Sonia's now giving me her verdict on the test results. She says, "I have taken in to all considerations your lifestyle and tablet medications that you are on. Your blood circulation to all parts of your hips and legs is fine."

I anxiously ask Sonia, "So what's making my legs and hip ache."

Sonia tells me, "It's the heart tablets that you are taking. In some people the heart tablets have a tendency to narrow the arteries as it has in your case Doug. This narrowing of your arteries is restricting your natural flow of blood to your hip and legs which, when you are walking a fair distance, your leg muscles are becoming starved of the natural oxygen supply which, in turn, causes your hip and legs to ache. As time passes on by and you keep on exercising and walking hopefully your aching hip and legs may resolve themselves."

I tell Sonia, "I have just recently been to see Mr Phil Batin, the Cardiologist, at this hospital, Pinderfields, and he told me exactly what you have just told me."

Sonia acknowledges with a nod. Sonia is now shaking my hand. As I am leaving, Sonia says, "Keep on rabbit catching as you always have but have a more leisurely approach to life," and on that I bid Sonia good day.

As time rolls on by (it's by now fifteen months since I had my double heart bypass operation), it's by now the month of March 2007, I can now tell you more about my aching legs and hip. I can now tell you my legs did resolve themselves quite significantly. I can now tell you that I can walk a fair distance without my calf muscles in my legs aching, except for when I climb a lot of steps. Take for example, all those steps at Leeds General Infirmary, from B Floor, Ground Floor, and climb up to F Floor, 5th Floor, which is 104 steps. That's when my calf muscles in my legs will ache, but I suppose that can be expected. I can now tell you about my aching left hip. That too has resolved itself a lot but not altogether. When I walk a fair distance I have a slight dull ache in my hip which I persevere and tolerate, so I think that's good news don't you? I can now tell you about my numbness in my left upper part of my breast. That has cleared itself altogether. I now have full feeling and sensitivity back again. The numbness in my leg, which is just above my ankle on the inside of my shin bone, that too has recovered a lot, but not altogether. It still feels slightly numb to the touch. Maybe give it a bit more time and that too may recover altogether. The scars down the middle of my breastbone, chest, and the full length of the inside of my leg have all about disappeared, nearly hardly noticeable.

A friend of mine, Graham, who I hadn't seen for quite a while saw the front of my shirt was open, he sees my chest scar and says, "Have you been cutting your chest."

I tell him I have had a double heart bypass operation. I show Graham the full length scar on my leg. Graham is captivated by the scars that he sees. He says, "I can hardly tell the scars were ever there at all, so that's a compliment from Graham to you and your medical team Mr Munsch.

I must admit I put my secret gypsy potion on my scar wounds which helps to heal at an incredible speed. This gypsy potion I speak of I acquired from an old friend of mine who they called Gypsy Benny, who alas now has died. It's many years ago now since Gypsy Benny showed me how to mix this secret Gypsy formula. We would go out into the grass fields and meadows. We would gather many certain herbs. Back at Gypsy Benny's encampment he would mix all these herbs together in a certain manner. He would brew them together in his brewing pot over the top of the open log burning fire. By the time the recipe was completed it came out of the brewing pot in a form of a jelly. This gypsy potion can now be smeared onto injured gallowers 'horses' which have bad cuts or gashes on them I have seen Gypsy Benny do this many times to injured gallowers and in a matter of no time the bad gashes on the gallowers would be healed over and never to be seen at all. Gypsy Benny swore me to secrecy and never to reveal the gypsy potion formula, and to this day I never have and never will.

I remember one particular incident happening which was many years ago now. I had many gallowers turned out in a field. I always had many gallowers which I dealt with at many horse fairs up and down the country. One of my gallowers had been racing and galloping itself around the field. It ran into a barbed wire fence and badly gashed its shoulder. The gash was so deep and severe I had to call in the vet. The vet came and stitched up the gallower's shoulder. When the vet leaves he says he will be back later to check on the gallower's progress of recovery. So, during the time of the vet's absence I would put my gypsy potion on the gallower's bad gash morning, noon and night. It healed over to perfection. The vet duly came back. He looked at the gallower's shoulder. I hear him mutter to himself. I see him shake his head. He now goes to the gallower's other shoulder. Again I hear him mutter to himself and again he shakes his head. The vet looks at me as I am holding the gallower. He says, "Doug, you will have to tell me where the injury is, I seem to have forgotten."

"There," as I point with my finger. The vet now scrutinises the area. There was nothing there to be seen of the scar. It had healed over completely and the hair had grown back to its normal self. I tell the vet I have been putting on my gypsy potion on the gallower's gash. The vet begged and prayed me to give him my gypsy potion formula. But alas I stayed, "Mum."

So that's what I put on my chest and leg scars, and now my friend Graham is just like the vet was. Graham is amazed at what he sees; my scar's hardly noticeable.

I can now tell you about my racing heartbeat. When I was in the Intensive Care Unit just after my operation with Diane, the Intensive Care Nurse, she was trying to control my racing heartbeat. Do you remember? Mr Munsch came to me that morning, his wise and comforting reassuring words were, "Your racing heartbeat will not hurt you Doug. Teach yourself to relax and accept your heartbeat. It's making you grow anxious. You have a fine healthy heartbeat there. You can teach yourself to slow your heartbeat down."

Those were the reassuring words I wanted to hear, especially coming from the tongue of a heart surgeon. Mr Munsch continued on to say, "Give me a little time and I will control your racing heartbeat with the right medication tablets that suits you."

So. putting those two together and now bringing in the showman who could slow down his heartbeat until it nearly stopped beating altogether, when I thought if the showman can slow his heartbeat down like that then surely I can slow my heartbeat and teach it to stop racing on. Do you remember all that?

Mr Munsch did get me on the right medication tablets, and that did stop my heartbeat racing on. To me this was a Godsend. All my life I have suffered my racing heartbeat and now my heart has succumbed and slowed down, "Phew."

I can now tell you, I did train my heart to go into deep slumber. Even though my heart was not now racing on, I could feel my heart fair pounding strong inside my chest. This is where my training comes in. I will get myself sitting or laying comfortably. I will put my mind fully on my heartbeat making and forcing it to go into slumber, and within a matter of no time at all. My heart has slowed down that much I cannot feel it beating at all. Simply amazing! Especially for me. I am now in a state of deep slumber. I am now in a state of contentment. This word 'contentment', in my mind, it's the finest word in the English language. It goes beyond compare. I would say there is not a single adult person in the whole of the world who is in complete contentment?

As I look back I see a long dusty road behind me. I say earlier in my story that we have had the misfortune of having to undergo major surgery of having to have a heart bypass, but I think we are the lucky ones. We have been diagnosed as having blocked up arteries, which could have proved fatal. There's many people out there who have blocked up arteries and they don't know they have. They could drop stone dead with a heart attack. We have now been given a second chance in life. We now have new blood vessels to our heart. I can now speak for myself and vouch for that.

I now, as I write my story (it's now 15 months after my double heart bypass) I live to tell my story. I am a new man again. I can now do everything that I always have done. I hope you have enjoyed reading my true to the fact story of my double heart bypass. We are the lucky ones. Good Luck.

Also available from the same author
THE LIFE AND TIMES OF A COUNTRY BOY

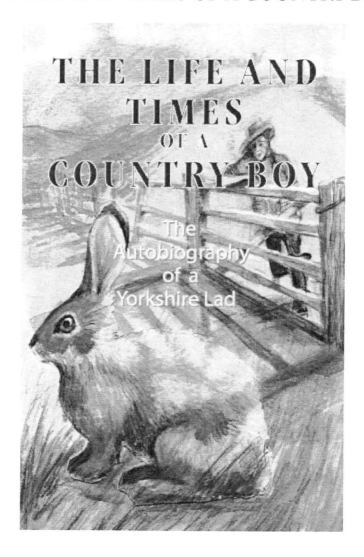

Available from all good book-selling websites and to order
through any reputable bookshop.
For the promptest response, order directly from the publisher:
www.upfrontbookshop.co.uk

Also available from the same author
THE LIFE AND TIMES OF A COUNTRY BOY

My own autobiography book, which was launched on to the worldwide market in the year of 2006, tells of my love for the fields and countryside beginning when I was only a lad of seven years old, my devilment of doing a bit of worldly poaching, getting myself chased many many times by the gamekeepers for poaching their rabbits, continuing on into adult life for my passionate love affair with nature's ways.

I tell of many characters I met along my way through life, spending many many years in the beautiful picturesque Yorkshire Dales. I tell of the true life story of a grouse moorland gamekeeper and his yearly cycle of the upkeep and the shooting of his large grouse moor.

With me being a little green-fingered, I taught myself the unique art of growing wild moorland heather high up on the hilltops, cultivated heather grows in the same manner.
My big secret now exposed, the growing of heather will now be revolutionized to the world.

And then there's my love of horse dealing among the Romany gypsies, travelling the country to all the horse fairs together with my beloved Appleby Horse Fair up in Westmoreland.

Now, as I look back over those distant bygone years of yesteryear, I leave a long dusty road behind me as I put pen to paper and write of my bygone years.

A hardy 206 pages of action-packed true-to-the fact stories.
Happy reading!

Available from all good book-selling websites and to order through any reputable bookshop.
For the promptest response, order directly from the publisher:
www.upfrontbookshop.co.uk